BEAT MENOPAUSE
NATURALLY

Contents

Acknowledgements...2
About the author 3
Shared story 4

Part – One – The Mechanisms

Chapter 1   Background to the Successful WNAS Program.......................6
Chapter 2   Menopause Symptoms Quantified 15
Chapter 3   Perimenopause meets Menopause....................................21
Chapter 4   Hormone Replacement Therapy – The Nitty Gritty...............35
Chapter 5   Nutrition & Hormone Function 40
Chapter 6   Detecting Nutritional Deficiencies 49
Chapter 7   Phytoestrogens – Mother Nature's Gift 52
Chapter 8   Heart Protection 60
Chapter 9   Healthy Bones 64
Chapter 10 Boosting Memory & Brain Power....................................71

Part –Two – The Solution

Chapter 11 Wean Yourself Off HRT 74
Chapter 12 Dietary & Lifestyle Recommendations 77
Chapter 13 The Benefits of Supplements.......................................81
Chapter 14 The Value of Exercise..88
Chapter 15 The Benefits of Relaxation...98
Chapter 16 Complementary Therapies 101
Frequently Asked Questions..103

Part – Three – The Tried & Tested Diet

Sample one week Phyto-Rich Menu..106
Recipe Corner..108
Phyto-Rich Food List 113
Nutrient Content of Food Lists 114
UK Directory of Soya-Rich Products 121
Australian Directory of Soya-Rich Products......................................122

Appendix

Medical References 123
Recommended Reading..124
WNAS Contact Details 124
Useful Contact Addresses 124
Links to useful Websites...124

Dedication

To Hilda Borkum, Mandy Farmer & Caroline Darke

with love and thanks for your true friendship

Acknowledgements

My first thanks must go to my patients over the last 19 years for providing me with the clinical evidence that our menopause programme is both effective and enjoyable. In particular, a big thank you goes to the patients who agreed to share their stories in this book in the unselfish hope that they could enlighten others.

My grateful thanks also to other researchers around the world who have shared their work and made it possible for us to devise a workable programme.

I am also grateful to Carys Glaberson and the team at the Women's Nutritional Advisory Service (WNAS) for keeping the show on the road while I was otherwise occupied, to Chesney for making this book look aesthetically pleasing, to Jane Garton for her help, support and editing skills and to Carys again for her hawkeye proofreading skills.

On the home front I'm enormously grateful to my children, Phoebe, Chesney, Hester and Simeon, for putting up with my utter preoccupation and being happy to share the computer with me. I'm also immensely grateful to Alan for being the chief cook and bottle washer while I slaved away over the hot keys.

Knowing the far-reaching health benefits as we do, we all think it was worth the effort and the sacrifice of our valuable leisure time.

Maryon Stewart

October 2003

www.beatmenopausenaturally.com

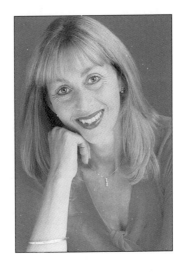

Maryon Stewart studied preventive dentistry and nutrition at St. George's Hospital in London and worked as a counsellor with nutritional doctors in England for four years. At the beginning of 1984 she set up the PMT Advisory Service, which has subsequently helped thousands of women world wide. In 1987 she launched the Women's Nutritional Advisory Service, which now provides broader help to women of all ages and as a result of her work was voted the 51st most influential woman in the UK in a Good Housekeeping Survey.

Maryon Stewart is the author of the best-selling books The Zest for Life Plan, The Phyto Factor, Cruising through The Menopause, No More PMS, now in its third edition, Beat Sugar Craving and Healthy Parents, Healthy Baby. She is the co-author of No More IBS, Beat PMS Cookbook and Every Woman's Health Guide and The Natural Health Bible. Her latest book, The Model Plan, was published while she was working as the nutritional consultant to the British Channel 4 programme Model Behaviour.

She has worked extensively on radio including on her own weekly radio programme on health and nutrition, has co-written several medical papers and has written for many national magazines and daily newspapers including the London Daily Mail, Daily Mirror and The London Express. She has also appeared on many TV programmes on all five channels. She was a regular contributor to Capital Woman, has done a series of Help Yourself programmes for Yorkshire TV and has also helped Anglia Television with their series Bodyworks. She has contributed to over 1000 radio programmes and was a regular contributor to House & Garden, Healthy Eating and the Sunday Express Magazine. She has been both advisor and contributor to Good Health Magazine, on the Expert Panel for Top Sante magazine and First Steps and is currently a consultant and regular contributor to Health & Fitness Magazine. She frequently lectures to both the public and the medical profession and runs a corporate health programme which educates employees about how to meet their body's nutritional needs. She is married to Dr. Alan Stewart with whom she has four children and lives in Lewes, Sussex.

maryon.stewart@naturalmenopause.com

Shared Story...

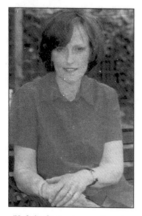

"I felt frumpy and ugly on HRT. Then I changed my diet and got my life back."

Helen, a university administrator, lives with her husband Eric and her two daughters Sally and Marie.

"I started getting menopausal symptoms when I was 45 and for years I felt I was living just half a life. I suffered tiredness to the point of collapse, excessive bloating, gas, breast tenderness, pain on ovulation and a gradual loss of interest in sex. I felt totally miserable.

The way I felt affected everything about my life, including my relationships with my family and friends. I used to have such a lot of energy, but found it more and more difficult to cope. That made me feel depressed and reduced me to tears. Eric was sympathetic, but at the same time he was bewildered by the way I had changed. Because I had lost so much self-confidence I couldn't open up to him, which made him feel shut out.

The girls would say, 'Oh, mother is in one of her funny moods again' or 'She's in a bad mood again'. It was very upsetting. I'd been to the doctor when the symptoms started and he did tests, but said I hadn't reached menopause. So I stuck it out for five years until the doctor finally thought HRT would help me.

"I felt very uneasy about it, partly because my mother had had breast cancer although, thankfully, she recovered. But the doctor said the benefits from HRT would far outweigh the risk of breast cancer in my case. He put me on Prempac C which is oestrogen and progestogen. For the first three months I felt wonderful - but then some of the symptoms returned. My stomach seemed to be ten times bigger, my clothes wouldn't fit, I felt frumpy and ugly. I had headaches and migraines. My skin became dry.

I hated the way I felt. I thought my natural periods might have stopped and I wanted to find out. In fact my periods didn't resume. Instead I had hot flushes about 12 times a day because of the oestrogen withdrawal. The heat would start in my stomach and envelop my whole body for several minutes. Afterwards I'd get this cold, clammy feeling, as if someone was walking over my grave. After two months I thought, 'I've had enough. I'm going to take control of my body'.

"I'd always been interested in self-help remedies. I had heard of the Women's Nutritional Advisory Service and went for a consultation in January. They put me on their Natural Menopause Programme, which included a change in diet, plus exercise and relaxation. They took me off wheat and caffeine. I was told to eat nuts, legumes and soya-based foods, plus fresh fruit and vegetables three times a day. I was prescribed multi-vitamins and supplements to overcome the hot flushes and guard against osteoporosis. Within a week I felt a difference. The hot flushes disappeared and I had tons more energy. I felt more positive, more relaxed and far happier.

"Eric is delighted to see the return of the wife he always knew, especially as my libido is returning. I know it's a cliché, but I really do feel like a new woman. I've got my life back and for the first time in years I feel positive about the future."

Chapter 1

Background to the Successful WNAS Programme

There has never been a better time for women wanting advice on natural menopause. The major international studies looking at the effects of Hormone Replacement Therapy (HRT) have now been aborted due to an increased incidence of serious medical problems, including coronary heart disease, stroke, thrombosis and both breast and ovarian cancer. The premature cessation of these trials across the world has sent shock waves through the menopausal community, especially among women who are currently taking HRT. Additionally, those who were debating whether to take hormones are now thinking twice before having their prescriptions filled.

At the Women's Nutritional Advisory Service we have been inundated with inquiries from women who are eager to come off HRT but are not sure how to go about it. They wonder if they should just stop their medication or should wean themselves off gradually. Well, the research shows that it's important to wean yourself off HRT very gradually, as sudden withdrawal is likely to result in a worsening of symptoms, especially hot flushes. There is now a wealth of evidence to support the scientifically based non-drug alternative approach to menopause.

Women can overcome the symptoms of menopause without having to resort to taking HRT. Nineteen years of helping women through their health problems at the Women's Nutritional Advisory Service (WNAS) allows me to put my hand on my heart and state with certainty that there is an effective scientifically based natural alternative available. Published research now clearly supports the fact that menopausal symptoms can be overcome without having to resort to HRT, while at the same time protect women from both heart disease and the bone thinning disease, osteoporosis, in the longer term. Despite this, the alternative approach is not widely known outside medical research circles, and is certainly not widely practised by doctors, largely because of their lack of education.

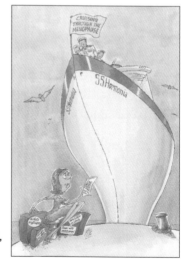

At the WNAS, over the last 16 years, we have pioneered an exceedingly simple, workable and enjoyable programme to help alleviate the symptoms of both perimenopause and menopause, no matter how severe. The success rate, within a matter of months, astounds most of the patients, and is a constant source of satisfaction to our team of health professionals. Although I get enormous satisfaction from helping individuals over their symptoms, the success brings with it a great deal of frustration. I constantly despair knowing that there is a workable alternative, based on sound research and extensive clinical practice and yet there are millions of women around the world who are left on what I call "the medical scrap heap", who have to fend for themselves not realising that there are simple and effective measures they can implement themselves which will alleviate their symptoms within a matter of weeks or months.

The purpose of 'Beat-Menopause-Naturally' is to explain clearly about the pros and cons of taking HRT and to spread the word about the workability of the WNAS programme to women everywhere thus enabling them to make informed choices and to remain in the driver's seat throughout menopause. I am sure you will agree that it is highly desirable to remain in good health for what may turn out to be the second half of your life. These days women are living so much longer, on average reaching their mid 80s, and in many cases far beyond. It is therefore vitally important that we become familiar with all the self-help measures that science provides, not just to overcome the distressing menopausal symptoms, but also to preserve the health of our heart, our bones and our mental well-being in the long-term.

To this day, HRT remains the treatment of choice for most doctors for both perimenopausal and menopausal women. This is mainly because, by their own admission, they lack education on the subject of nutrition as undergraduates and the majority of their post-graduate education comes from the pharmaceutical companies, many of whom are the producers of HRT. This may be fine for the women who feel happy and well taking HRT, however, research shows that up to two-thirds of women who try HRT come off it within the first year because of side effects or dissatisfaction. There are also women

Table 1. Recommendations from nutritional and patient: a doctor's responsibility

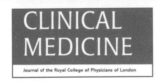

1. All doctors should be aware of nutritional problems and how to manage them. Every doctor should recognise that proper nutritional care is fundamental to good clinical practice

who cannot take HRT for a variety of medical reasons, and indeed there are women for whom HRT is not an option they would willingly consider. Despite this, according to the results of our latest survey of 1000 physicians in general practice, there are very few doctors who are equipped with the knowledge to provide scientifically based alternative advice. So even now, despite the wealth of published papers on the non-drug approach to menopause, many women are either locked into taking HRT whether they like it or not, or alternatively are left to fend for themselves.

Repeated WNAS surveys on menopausal women constantly confirm the fear and confusion they experience about the changes and symptoms that accompany menopause and the prospect of becoming a victim of the bone thinning disease, osteoporosis. These days we often encounter conflicting reports about the pros and cons of HRT and the workability of alternative approaches, both in scientific journals and the media. 'Beat Menopause Naturally' is designed to put an end to the confusion by presenting the scientific evidence in easily understandable terms. Once you have the facts at your fingertips, you will be armed with all the information you need in order to make an informed choice about how to manage your menopause.

The WNAS Programme makes it all so simple...

Over the last 16 years we have helped thousands of women through their perimenopause and even more to overcome their menopausal symptoms. Our programme has become increasingly successful in recent years, as science has provided us with even more workable tools. In 'Beat Menopause Naturally' I have presented the "secrets" behind the WNAS programme, so that you can devise a programme to help yourself through perimenopause and overcome those menopausal symptoms and even wean yourself off HRT. As you work your way through the book you will discover that the WNAS programme we have devised over the years consists mainly of the following:

● Making specific dietary changes including:
  - improving the nutrient content of your diet and removing foods that may impede the absorption of good nutrients
  - removing from the diet foods that will worsen hot flushes and night sweats
  - including foods in the diet that are rich in naturally occurring oestrogens, known as phytoestrogens, a gift from Mother Nature, allowing us to supplement natural oestrogen on a daily basis.
● Taking nutritional supplements including vitamins, minerals, herbs and phytoestrogen rich supplements which have proved their value in clinical trials

- Moderate weight bearing exercise to stimulate the brain chemistry and to help keep both our heart and our bones in a healthy condition
- A regular relaxation programme that, research shows, dramatically reduces hot flushes and helps to keep you feeling in control.

The programme also includes menu plans both for meat eaters and vegetarians and some delicious recipes to incorporate into your repertoire if you enjoy cooking. If you are not one of life's devoted cooks, or don't have much time to spend in the kitchen, then you will enjoy the numerous fast, but nutritious, options which take very little time to prepare, but still provide you with the necessary nutrients.

CASE HISTORY 1

Hillary, 49 from London, came to the WNAS with severe menopausal symptoms

BEFORE:	AFTER ONE MONTH ON THE WNAS PHYTOESTROGEN-RICH PROGRAMME:
✘ Hot and cold flushes during the day	✔ All hot and cold flushes had completely stopped
✘ Insomnia	
✘ Depression	✔ Less anxious
✘ Digestive problems	✔ Losing weight steadily
✘ Sudden weight gain	✔ Sleeping well
✘ A feeling of losing her grip on life	✔ Exceedingly happy!

Is menopause primarily hormonal?

Until recently, the widely-held view was that virtually all the symptoms of menopause could be explained on the basis of a failure by the ovaries. Such a view was strongly supported by the experience and testimony of many women who had taken HRT and experienced dramatic relief from many of their symptoms. While there is a strong relationship between some menopausal symptoms and the falling levels of the hormone oestrogen, because we are extremely complex animals, it stands to reason that there are other biological mechanisms at play. These should not only be considered but should also open the door to alternative and more natural solutions to HRT, and we will be examining this issue shortly.

CASE HISTORY 2

Angela, 49, from the West Midlands, came to the WNAS for an alternative to HRT

BEFORE:

✘ Hot flushes – "on fire"
✘ Headaches
✘ Fatigue
✘ Constipated
✘ Gained 21 pounds on HRT

AFTER FOUR MONTHS ON THE WNAS PHYTOESTROGEN-RICH PROGRAMME:

✔ All hot flushes gone
✔ No headaches
✔ No constipation
✔ Lost weight – 11 pounds
✔ Feels like she is back in the driver's seat!

Why do women suffer at menopause?

To understand what happens to the body at the time of menopause it is necessary to go back in time to the child bearing years. Many physical demands are placed upon us in these early years, which can result in poor health prospects when not met. At the WNAS, we know from our own research on women of child-bearing age with premenstrual syndrome (PMS), that between 50 and 80 per cent of them have a shortage of an important mineral called magnesium and other nutrients like B vitamins, iron, zinc and essential fatty acids are often in short supply.

The importance of nutrients

Let's use magnesium as an example. It's needed for:

● Normal brain chemical metabolism

● Normal hormone function

● Smooth muscle control (both the uterus and the gut are smooth muscles)

It follows, therefore, that a shortage of magnesium alone can influence both physical and mental well-being, all aspects of our menstrual cycle, and our intestinal function.

Extra nutrient demands are also placed on women's bodies during pregnancy and even more so when breast-feeding. Mother Nature in her wisdom ensures that the growing baby gets all the nutrients needed for development, which means they go sailing across the placenta and through the breast milk, often leaving the mother in a poor nutritional state.

As years go by, levels of some nutrients in women's bodies reduce naturally. By the time we reach menopause we are often in a nutritionally depleted state, effectively firing on two cylinders instead of four. Since menopause is such a major transition in a woman's life, the body needs to be in good shape to ensure a smooth passage, and because of these nutritional imbalances, many women can experience uncomfortable and disturbing symptoms. For instance, the hot flushes that are experienced at the time of menopause are simply the result of brain chemistry attempting to kick-start the ovaries back into function at the time when our natural oestrogen levels have fallen as a result of dwindling ovarian function. Eating foods that contain naturally occurring oestrogen and improving nutritional status through diet and lifestyle can have a positive influence on brain chemistry. As a result hot flushes and night sweats dramatically subside.

Later in this book you'll read about the survey we conducted with 2003 women who had recently been through menopause. We found their symptoms broke down into three separate categories. The first group, perhaps the most obvious, were the oestrogen-withdrawal symptoms: hot flushes, night sweats, dry vagina and insomnia. These symptoms were directly related to falling oestrogen levels in the body.

We call the remaining two groups 'physical symptoms' – aches, pains, migraines, headaches, irritable bowel syndrome and fatigue – and the 'mental symptoms' – panic attacks, palpitations, mood swings, aggression and depression. Most interestingly, the survey revealed that both the 'physical' and the 'mental' symptoms were more related to dietary and lifestyle inadequacies than they were to falling oestrogen levels in the body. Another survey conducted on 200 menopause patients in 1997 echoed this. It showed that the physical and mental symptoms were more prevalent at the time of menopause than the oestrogen withdrawal symptoms.

This was an extraordinary finding and lies at the heart of our advice about menopause and its treatment. Now that we can appreciate the symptoms experienced at menopause are not necessarily all to do with falling oestrogen levels, our expectations of HRT, as a result of its media image, may be too high. HRT is designed mainly to counteract the oestrogen-withdrawal symptoms rather than the 'physical' and 'mental' symptoms we have now identified. The WNAS programme, however, aims to address all these groups of symptoms effectively.

One audit on patients who have been through our programme showed that 90 per cent of women feel that their menopause symptoms are under control within four months (Group 1, oestrogen-withdrawal symptoms) and a similar percentage reported having overcome 'physical' and 'mental' symptoms within the same time period.

When we restore the balance and put back in the body what time and nature have taken out, it seems to have a normalising effect on brain chemistry and hormone function. It is similar to turning the factory lights back on. It is almost as if the women return to their pre-menopausal condition.

Having treated tens of thousands of patients over the years at the WNAS I have witnessed many wonderful transformations as women regain their quality of health, confidence and self-esteem. Our 'case histories', who have generously shared their stories with us in this book, are a few typical examples.

Jo's Story

Jo De Lisle was a retired teacher from Kent who lived with her husband and two sons. She was recovering from a nervous breakdown following extreme harrassement she had experienced in the workplace. She was suicidal and said she was suffering with self-disgust.

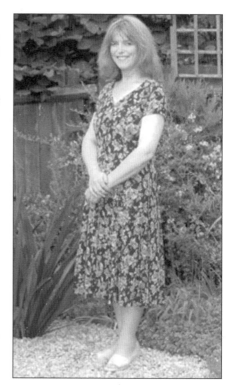

"I first experienced symptoms of menopause four years ago. My periods became very frequent and I began to have hot flushes. I took early retirement from work following a very unpleasant situation that got out of hand. I felt as if I was suffering with bereavement, grieving the loss of myself. I had terrible hot flushes and mood swings for which my doctor prescribed HRT.

Almost immediately, I started gaining weight – 70 pounds in all, which was four dress sizes! I had headaches on HRT which seemed to last all day and all night and what felt like constant PMS. I had gas, bloating and constipation and an obsession with chocolate. Some days I would forget to eat anything except chocolate. My friend phoned me one day and told me that she had seen Maryon Stewart who had helped her overcome her severe menopausal symptoms. She lent me one of Maryon's books and told me to make an appointment to see her. I was in such a state I didn't even get around to making an appointment. I then went through a period of feeling suicidal for three weeks and my husband finally cracked as he couldn't cope. He hit out at our 15-year-old son and it ended with both my sons and my husband crying. I knew I had to seek help.

Maryon listened carefully to my tale of woe and gave me a great deal of reassurance. I wasn't at all convinced but realized I had to give her recommendations a try. I came off the HRT and followed the programme as best I could. Within six weeks I felt like a different person. I wasn't spaced out any more and realized that I had lost three years of my life. I had no more panic attacks or depression and felt like I had managed to take control of my body once more.

As the months passed I felt happier and more positive than I had for years and the weight started to fall off. I feel calm, happy to the point of feeling bubbly and people I know walk by me in the street as my physical appearance is so completely different. I feel like I have found a new me. I honestly never thought I would live to see the day when I could lead a normal happy life again and I am so very grateful."

Jo and the many other case histories who have kindly agreed to appear in this book will assure you that you are not suffering alone and will give you confidence that the end of your symptoms is in sight. Realistically, you will need to invest in yourself for the next four to six months in order to help yourself back to good health. According to our research, the degree to which you follow the recommendations is directly related to how much better you will feel. Once you have read through the book and worked out the programme to follow, stick to it like superglue!

If you feel you can't manage alone and would like some extra help or advice then you will find the WNAS contact details at the end of the book. It's never too early to improve your general health and to work towards preventing osteoporosis, so as you approach menopausal age, even if you are symptom-free, work out a diet that you would find enjoyable, using the guidelines given later in the book, together with a moderate exercise and nutritional supplement regime. If you start in time you might even sail through the menopause without noticing it!

Whether you are approaching perimenopause, currently in the throes of menopause, or have just emerged from it, you will need to read the first parts of the book and then go on to work out your tailor-made programme from the guidelines in the second part of the book. You will also find daily menus and delicious recipes to try as well as notes on the nutritional content of food. This will help you choose the foods you like, knowing that they are rich in essential vitamins and minerals.

Finding the programme that your body thrives on is a voyage of discovery that you need only make once. It's a voyage that both you and your family will undoubtedly be glad you undertook as you once again experience good health and well-being.

I wish you the very best of luck and would love to hear about your success as a result of following my recommendations. You can email me at the following address <u>maryon.stewart@naturalmenopause.com</u>

Chapter 2

Menopause Symptoms Quantified

Menopause brings with it rapid changes and unwanted symptoms which often disrupt life and result in utter misery. Up to 75 per cent of women can experience one or more of the effects of menopause such as frequent hot flushes during the day and sweats at night leaving them exhausted, disorientated and despondent. Vaginal dryness and reduced libido can wreck sex lives and repeated insomnia can make women wonder whether life as they knew it is over. The good news is that these symptoms can be overcome naturally with the only side effect being that you feel more like your old self and in some cases, a whole lot better.

> **Fact**
>
> Menopause definition - Date of last natural menstruation.
> It is a date not a duration.

What Are The Symptoms?

A survey conducted by the Women's Nutritional Advisory Service (WNAS) of 500 women who had recently gone through their menopause discovered that there were three main groups of symptoms that occur at the time of menopause. Only one group, however, is directly related to falling oestrogen levels. The other two groups have more to do with dietary and lifestyle inadequacies.

1. Oestrogen withdrawal symptoms

These are predominantly:

- hot flushes
- night sweats
- vaginal dryness
- loss of libido
- urinary symptoms
- difficulties with intercourse

2. Physical symptoms

These consist of:

- aches and pains

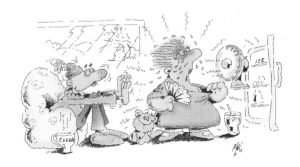

- irritable bowel syndrome
- constipation and fatigue
- migraines and headaches

3. Mental symptoms

These include:

- anxiety
- panic attacks
- irritability
- mood swings
- depression and confusion
- memory loss

What is not widely appreciated is that HRT, the most widely prescribed solution by doctors, is only aiming at the oestrogen withdrawal group and may not necessarily help the physical and mental symptoms.

From research conducted on several groups of women of child bearing age suffering with premenstrual syndrome, it was discovered that minerals like magnesium, iron and the B vitamins are often in short supply. This affects the efficiency of brain chemistry and hormone function. Menopause, which can test physical and emotional reserves, is a substantial transition for the body. If the body is not firing on all cylinders because of existing dietary inadequacies and a stressful lifestyle, it is more likely that menopausal symptoms could be more of a problem.

Shared Experiences

Like many things in life, menopause has its pros and cons. It brings with it a 'minestrone' of emotions. While most women are delighted that they no longer have a monthly period, many of the other signs and symptoms of menopause are usually not quite so welcome. At the WNAS we undertook another survey of 500 women going through menopause to see how they really felt about this phase in their lives.

Menopause 500 survey 2002

In the summer of 2002 we analysed a survey of 500 women who had recently gone through their menopause to see which were the most common symptoms suffered. It was interesting to note that there are many other symptoms apart from hot flushes, night sweats, insomnia and dry vagina that are causing major problems at the time of menopause. It was also a revelation to discover that nearly twice as many women in this sample who were on HRT lost their libido compared with those that had not chosen the hormone option.

PHYSICAL SYMPTOMS SAMPLE OF 500 WOMEN

	% Who suffer
• Hot flushes	74%
• Night sweats	70%
• Disturbed sleep	73%
• Poor concentration and memory	72%
• Reduced libido	65%
• Aches and pains	64%
• Vaginal dryness	53%

Other complaints included:

• Headaches	47%
• Constipation	42%
• Bad breath	26%

MENTAL SYMPTOMS SAMPLE OF 500 WOMEN	
	% Who suffer
● Anxiety	59%
● Confusion	58%
● Loss of confidence	55%
● Irritability	54%
● Depression	49%

Menopause 2003 Survey

In January 2003, at the WNAS we analysed a survey sample of 2003 women going through menopause.

Menopausal Symptoms

The most common menopausal symptoms were:

Disturbed sleep pattern	84%
Hot flushes	83%
Night sweats	80%
Poor concentration and memory	72%
Aches and pains	72%
Reduced libido	64%
Depression	64%
Headaches	60 %
Vaginal dryness	59%

Alternatives to HRT

60% of all the women surveyed had visited their doctor for advice on treatment for menopause related problems

And 17% of these had been offered an alternative to HRT.

Many women had sought alternatives themselves and typically such women had tried two or three different alternatives. The popularity of these and self-assessed benefit are presented in the table below.

Popularity of Self-help measures

	Total	No Help	Some Help	Very Helpful	Total Help
Multivitamins	1202	39%	53%	8%	61%
Vitamin E	842	35%	55%	10%	65%
Minerals	691	36%	55%	9%	64%
Isoflavone supplements	397	21%	59%	20%	79%
Homeopathy	373	38%	52%	10%	62%
Acupuncture	116	41%	40%	19%	59%
Ginseng	366	48%	44%	8%	52%
Dong Quai	274	39%	50%	11%	61%
Reflexology	191	33%	55%	12%	67%
Yoga	331	27%	55%	18%	73%

Women were also asked what further changes they might be willing to make to try and control their symptoms. The results are presented in the table below.

Acceptability of treatments for the control of menopausal symptoms

	Very willing	Moderately willing	Not willing
Modify diet	56%	42%	2%
Use natural products	77%	22%	1%
Relaxation therapy	59%	36%	5%
Physical exercise	54%	42%	4%
Take HRT	14%	36%	50%
Take other medication	13%	50%	37%

67% of women surveyed preferred to manage their menopause naturally. The most popular preferred approach would be to use a natural product, presumably in tablet or other easy to administer form. Relaxation therapy, increased physical exercise and modification of diet were very acceptable to over 50% of women. This group already had a high background prevalence of stress (70% considered themselves to be stressed).

● In particular, isoflavone-rich supplements were self-reported as being of some help or very helpful to 79% of those who had tried them

It would appear from this survey that an increasing number of women are either reluctant to take HRT or are becoming increasingly aware of actual or potential side effects. They are eager to look for alternatives and are willing to consider a diverse number of alternatives that may help to control not only their immediate menopause related symptoms but that may also bring health benefits in the longer term.

Fact

Perimenopause definition: The time of change leading up to actual menopause, and usually lasts about five years

---

Chapter 3

Perimenopause Meets Menopause

Menopause often brings with it a set of new symptoms that have never been experienced before. Menopause may well coincide with a number of other health factors and the degree of severity may well be associated with the timing of the symptoms and whether you have had a hysterectomy.

Let us first look at what has been happening in your body prior to menopause.

The normal menstrual cycle

Approximately each month, until we reach perimenopause, which is the five years before menopause when the body begins going through changes, under normal circumstances our ovaries produce an egg ready for fertilisation. This happens under the stimulus and direction of hormones produced by the pituitary gland which is situated at the base of the brain, a few inches behind our eyes. It produces many hormones to control the thyroid gland in the neck, the adrenal glands in the abdomen and the ovaries. It has been likened to the conductor of a hormonal orchestra. It controls hormone output by these glands on a day-to-day and even minute-to-minute basis. The ovary, for its part, provides two main elements - the eggs which come pre-formed as Graafian follicles (named after their discoverer) and the theca or substance of the ovary in which the tiny follicles are embedded, which is responsible for the production of the female sex hormones, oestrogen and progesterone.

The ovary has a limited supply of eggs all of which were formed in the womb before your own birth – hence the importance of your mother's health and diet during pregnancy. Each month several follicles are stimulated to develop by a hormone from the pituitary called, appropriately, follicle stimulating hormone or FSH. Usually one follicle, occasionally more, matures to a point where an egg is released, an event that normally takes place in the middle of the cycle. The egg is released as a result of a small rise in FSH and a very large surge of a second hormone from the pituitary called luteinising hormone or LH.

In the first part of the cycle the ovaries are also busy producing oestrogen, which encourages the lining of the womb to thicken so that it might be ready, should fertilisation take place. Oestrogen levels continue at a moderate level after ovulation and are joined by the second female sex hormone, progesterone. The follicle in the ovary produces this after the egg has been released and reaches a substantial peak around day 21 in the cycle. It then falls away unless fertilisation takes place and the rapid fall in the level of progesterone causes the lining of the womb to be shed in the form of a period.

So these two key hormones from the pituitary, FSH and LH, dictate the events in the ovary in terms of whether ovulation will take place or not and how much of the hormones, oestrogen and progesterone, will be in circulation.

Timing

There is a substantial variation in the timing of menopause. Most women will have their last natural period somewhere between the ages of 45 and 55, with an average of between 50 and 51 years. Interestingly, there has been little change in the time of the onset of symptoms over the last 100 years and even in the Middle Ages 50 years was about the norm. The age at the onset of menopause varies between cultures. Black women, for example, tend to experience an earlier menopause than white women in the US, and it can be nearly ten years earlier in malnourished women from developing countries. Nutrition, chronic infection and chronic illness in developing countries are factors that need to be taken into consideration.

Just why is there such a divergence in the Western population? Several studies have been conducted to look at what determines the age of menopause. By far the biggest determinant of an early menopause is smoking. It seems the more you smoke, the sooner your periods cease, adding to the toxic effects of smoking and providing yet another reason to stop or cut down. Heavy smokers can reach menopause two years earlier than their non-smoking counterparts.

Other lesser factors that have been linked to a slightly earlier menopause are — never having had children; possibly being short or underweight and possibly finishing your last pregnancy before the age of 28.

Just because your periods begin early does not mean that you will finish your periods earlier. It was once thought that an early start to periods meant that menopause would be later, but even this theory has been discounted.

As the ovaries running out of eggs mainly determine the cessation of our periods, it would not be surprising if the factors present at the time your eggs were being formed are relevant. Since this takes place before you were born, perhaps what was going on during your mother's pregnancy needs to be considered. Astonishingly, when the ovaries are developing some five to seven million follicles are formed by the fifth month of pregnancy. By the time the baby is born this has fallen to around two million and continues to fall thereafter. Mother Nature is already sorting out the wheat from the chaff.

It is now known that the female offspring of smokers are more likely to have difficulty getting pregnant, perhaps because their ovaries have taken a knock. Low birth-weight, being premature or severe illness of the mother during pregnancy might also be factors. We will have to see what future research reveals. Nutrition may well be a factor, too, as smoking adversely affects the levels of many nutrients. Smokers tend to eat less well that non-smokers and, as we shall see, there are a number of essential nutrients that influence hormone metabolism, hormone problems and the function of the ovaries.

The story doesn't end there. During perimenopause, the time just prior to the last actual period, the rate of follicle loss increases in line with the rise in the level of pituitary hormones. It might be possible that anything that increases the sensitivity of the ovary to respond to these stimulating hormones, such as the balance of certain nutrients, can help to delay the final day. This might account for the fact that so many women who have consulted us after going into an early menopause, in their late 30s or early 40s, have begun to menstruate regularly again after following our programme for a few months.

Zoe's Story

ZOE McKIRDY, 30, is single and works as a nanny in Hastings, East Sussex. When Hodgkin's lymphoma, a form of cancer was diagnosed, chemotherapy and radiation brought on the symptoms of menopause in her early 20's. She made dramatic changes to her diet and is delighted that doctors have found her ovaries are once more active.

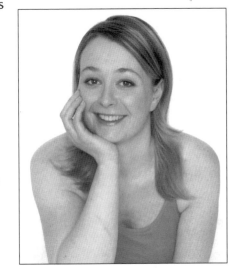

"My problem began in my early teens. I had what I thought was a muscular ache in my shoulder and my parents took me to see an osteopath. I thought it was caused by sleeping in a draft, but after a few months the pain wasn't getting better. My mother took me to our doctor and he sent me to the hospital to have an X-ray and CT scan. A biopsy diagnosed the illness.

Everything happened so quickly. I didn't have much time to feel scared. In many ways I think it was worse for my parents. I had nine months chemotherapy and lost my hair. Between the treatments I started college training to be a nanny. I was determined to get on with life. I never thought it would kill me.

One of the most devastating effects of the chemo, apart from losing my hair, was the effect on my reproductive cycle. It triggered a dramatic premature menopause. My periods became erratic and I suffered awful mood swings. I was horrible; really bad tempered, grouchy and snappy.

I would go months without a period and then have two heavy ones one after the other. It became worse in my 20s when I also began to get night sweats and hot flushes. My body felt like it was going mad.

My mother suggested that I see menopause expert Maryon Stewart. She had been seeing her for years and following her diet and exercise plan to cope with her menopause.

I was sceptical at first, but within a month I was converted. Maryon told me to stop eating wheat and gluten and to start taking a host of mineral and vitamin supplements. I cut out bread, fatty foods, red meat and caffeine and I take magnesium, multi-vitamins and isoflavone rich supplements.

A few years ago the doctors told me I'd have difficulty conceiving as my ovaries were shrivelled, but a recent scan revealed that my ovaries are healthy and active. The nurse said: 'Whatever you're doing, keep doing it.' I am confident I will be able to have children. I have lost a lot of weight, I no longer have PMS or menopause symptoms and the irritable bowel syndrome has gone too. I feel great and am so pleased that I am back in control of my life. I am very grateful to the WNAS".

Perimenopause

You may not have grasped the fact that there is another phase in your life that comes before menopause known as perimenopause. Peri simply means around, and it seems that changes that occur during perimenopause can begin from anything up to five years before menopause strikes.

For most women, ovulation is a regular event between the ages of 20 and 40. From approximately the age of 40 onwards, the supply of Graafian follicles begins to run out. There may be cycles in which the level of oestrogen is slightly reduced. The pituitary senses this and increases its release of FSH to stimulate the tiring ovary but more slowly, so that the time between cycles becomes longer and shorter. Progesterone levels will fall as ovulation does not always occur.

The second hormone from the pituitary gland, LH also rises a little later on. As oestrogen levels fall to very low levels the lining of the womb loses its main source of stimulation and periods cease. Levels of FSH and LH remain high for several years as they continue to live in hope before they finally get the message and subsequently fall away.

Most of us are unprepared for perimenopause. For some it simply brings a degree of unpredictability into our lives, during which time we experience irregular periods and

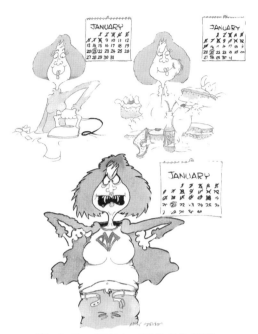

THE PMT JEKYLL & HYDE MONSTER

some periods may be lighter, while others become heavier, with perhaps the odd hot flash or night sweat. Mood swings often occur and a degree of depression is common. Those least fortunate women may experience a worsening of their PMS symptoms at this time as well as constant mood swings and more black days than they care to count.

When PMS meets menopause

It's bad luck if your PMS bumps into the start of your menopause symptoms and you have the worst of both worlds. It is a common problem, but fortunately one that can be sorted out effectively within a few months. Numerous studies reveal that the occurrence of cyclical physical and mental symptoms that are present just before the arrival of a period and diminish or disappear with or shortly after its arrival are at their most prevalent in the 30-something age group. So what are they doing here in a book on menopause? Well, for some women PMS never quite goes away and can even become worse in the perimenopausal phase. This is due to the hormonal instability at this time.

This, and other hormone-related factors, have caused many researchers in the past to attribute PMS to a lack or an excess of any hormone you care to mention. The medical profession does not speak with one voice on this matter. More critical research, however, has found no consistent hormonal abnormality in the majority of PMS sufferers but a more modern understanding is to ascribe the cause of PMS to an undue sensitivity on the part of the sufferer to the normal hormonal changes that take place in the last half of the cycle. Now this makes it much easier to see how PMS might fit in with some women's perimenopausal experience.

Maureen's Story

Maureen Gallagher had remedied her PMS with my help ten years ago. She had stayed in good shape for many years but she became perimenopausal in her early 40s when she was also experiencing lots of stress. She came back for help as she felt she had lost control.

"I had been coasting along nicely for years since sorting out my severe PMS in the early 1990s. I suppose I got complacent along the way as things were going so well. I didn't really pay much attention to myself as I was too busy dealing with needs of my family. My teenage daughter was going through a 'wild child' phase and my husband had a nervous breakdown. I managed to cope with it all but I was in a bit of a daze one day when I got knocked off my bicycle by a car and it was only then when I had to take time off from work to recover that I realized how badly I had let things slip. My periods had become irregular and very heavy, leaving me feeling drained. My mood swings and depression had returned and I was feeling incredibly tired.

I got back in touch with Maryon and completed a new questionnaire and diet diary. I knew she would provide me with the encouragement and advice I needed to deal with my current situation. And sure enough she did. I should have expected an early menopause with hindsight, as my mother started hers in her early 40s too. I made all the changes to my diet that Maryon suggested and changed my supplement regime. I got back to exercising and I retrained and qualified as a special needs assistant.

My periods are much more regular now and the flooding has stopped. I am far less stressed and have coped really well with my daughter's teenage pregnancy and supported her and the rest of the family with lots of new-found energy.

I do feel like I am back in control of my life and I feel much more alive and energetic. I am fully briefed about how to get through perimenopause in good health and much more at peace with myself. As usual I am very grateful to Maryon for all her caring efforts".

Most women who suffer from PMS do not enjoy the hormonal roller coaster. Furthermore, the most successful treatments include anything that effectively switches off the ovaries. No working ovaries means no PMS! Oestrogen implants work like magic, producing a near-religious experience for some women. But sadly, the benefit may not last because the body adjusts to a new hormonal balance and the natural cycle re-imposes itself.

Our own substantial experience and that of others who have also published their results is that PMS can be helped with a change of diet, the use of certain nutritional supplements and physical exercise. These factors can all influence female hormone function, nervous-system chemistry, general well-being and physical fitness. They can do so in a far more gentle and as effective a way as the 'best' hormonal treatment.

In one of the surveys I mentioned earlier we also looked at the relationship between previous PMS suffering and current menopausal symptoms. The difficulty with this sort of question is that the person's perception of the past may be influenced by their current state of health.

There did seem to be a moderate connection between the severity of past premenstrual symptoms and some current menopausal symptoms. This held true for symptoms of depression, anxiety, confusion and insomnia in particular, whereas physical symptoms, such as hot flushes and night sweats showed only a minor degree of association with past PMS.

It would, therefore, seem that symptoms that are mainly attributable to oestrogen withdrawal, such as hot flushes, are not greatly influenced by a history of PMS. 'Mental' symptoms, however, do seem to show some kind of continuity. It is not possible from the questions we asked to discern how much of this was due to psychological problems, or hormonal or other health problems.

As diet and lifestyle seem to make such a big difference to many women's PMS this is good news for many menopausal women going through similar mood changes at the time of menopause.

The normal menopause

The last actual period denotes the date of menopause itself. This can only be determined with hindsight, usually after there have been no periods for at least six months in a woman of suitable age, with typical symptoms or with hormonal evidence of menopause. The most common test is to measure FSH, LH and oestrogen levels in the blood.

During the time just prior to menopause there is considerable instability, with all these hormonal changes occurring. Not surprisingly this is the time when symptoms can be most troublesome, especially if you already suffer from premenstrual syndrome.

Sarah's Story

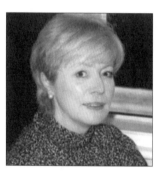

Sarah Andrews is a housewife from Surrey who lived with her husband and daughter. She was suffering with severe anxiety and panic attacks and a terrible lack of confidence and was very frightened about the way she felt. She said that she felt like a shadow of her former self.

" I first experienced symptoms of menopause two and a half years ago. My periods became very frequent and heavy and I had terrible gas, bloating and constipation and extreme cravings for savoury food. I felt very lethargic and had gained 14 pounds. My doctor suggested HRT tablets. Almost immediately, I started gaining weight and felt grotty. I tried to stop taking the HRT but within a few days I felt suicidal. I read an article in the Mail on Sunday about Maryon Stewart's work at the WNAS and I then went out and bought one of her books. I was relieved to discover that there might be a solution to my problems so I contacted the Women's Nutritional Advisory Service and made an appointment to see Maryon in her Lewes clinic. Maryon designed a programme for me to follow and helped wean me off the HRT tablets.

Within a month many of my symptoms had disappeared and I was feeling amazingly better. The gas, bloating and constipation were gone and I was feeling less irritable and I lost seven pounds. I came off HRT and had a period with much less PMS than usual.

As the months passed I felt happier and more positive than I had for years and the weight started to fall off. I made a big mistake though as I got complacent. I stopped following the diet strictly and the panic attacks and anxiety began to return. I went back to see Maryon for a review and her enthusiasm gave me the incentive to get back on track. It's been over a year now. I have lost weight and am able to really enjoy my life to the fullest".

Hysterectomy

Christine Hicks

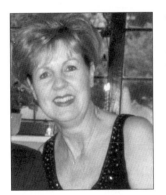

Christine Hicks, a mother of two from just outside London, was 52 when she first came to see me. She had a radical hysterectomy and a mastectomy three months previously after which she haemorrhaged badly. She was suffering severe hot flushes, night sweats, insomnia and very low hemoglobin. She was feeling very poorly as you can imagine and was desperate to find help as she was not a candidate for HRT because of her history of cancer and a pulmonary embolism 15 years earlier.

"I was at a very low ebb when I went to see Maryon Stewart after reading two of her books. I had been through a series of medical upheavals not least of which was the burst valve following a breast reconstruction, which resulted in three further operations in quick succession. Having had nine anaesthetics in less than two years and with extremely low iron levels I was finding it difficult to lead anything that resembled a normal life. I have a wonderful husband and two lovely daughters and everything to live for, but I felt like I was just clinging on to life.

The hot flushes and night sweats were getting progressively worse since starting on the Tamoxifen which I knew I would have to keep taking, no matter what. My fatigue from lack of iron was further compounded by my severely disrupted night's sleep due to the constant night sweats.

Maryon was very reassuring and designed a plan for me to follow which involved making dietary changes and taking some supplements. I wasn't fit enough to exercise even though I used to go regularly to our local gym. I followed the suggested recommendations and by my first follow-up appointment, which was four weeks later, I was feeling quite a bit better with more energy and feeling more like I could control my own destiny. I had been suffering with irritable bowel syndrome since the cancer was diagnosed, but once I got established on the programme the pain and diarrhoea disappeared. I remember on the day of that appointment I only had one hot flash, which was a dramatic improvement.

Within three months I was feeling really well. I was sleeping well, and the flushes during the day and night were a thing of the past. I had lost seven pounds without trying and no longer had the chocolate cravings I had been plagued with all my life. I managed to really enjoy an active holiday to celebrate our 30th wedding anniversary and I organised two weddings for both our daughters.

I am extremely grateful for the help and support Maryon has given me as I feel that as a result I can now lead a normal life once again."

Hysterectomy is the surgical removal of the womb and is one of the most common operations performed. Some 20,000 take place in the UK each year and approximately a staggering 600,000 are performed each year in the US. It involves the removal of the womb, either through an incision in the abdomen or, in about 25 per cent of cases, by removal through the vagina. A total hysterectomy just removes the womb including the cervix or neck of the womb. Sometimes the ovaries, which are at either side of the uterus, are also removed together with neighbouring tissues; this is called a radical hysterectomy. The ovaries may need to be removed if they are diseased with large cysts, endometriosis or cancer.

Studies have revealed great variations in the frequency with which hysterectomies are performed, especially in different regions of the US. Though there is agreement about the need for hysterectomy in women with uterine cancer, there is not much agreement about its need for non-cancerous reasons such as fibroids, heavy periods and pelvic pain. Recently, two detailed American publications have looked at the reasons why hysterectomies are performed and their outcome. Data collected by the National Centre for Health Statistics in Atlanta revealed the rate of just under 600,000 hysterectomies per year for the years 1988-90. The overall rate per year was just below six hysterectomies for every 1,000 women rising to ten in the 30 to

54 year age group. The overall rate was slightly higher in black women compared to white. The most common reason was uterine fibroids followed by endometriosis, prolapse and cancer among others. Fibroids were listed as the reason twice as commonly in whites when compared with blacks. The ovaries were removed in 50 per cent of the operations and this became more likely with increasing age. However, oophorectomy, the medical term for the removal of the ovaries, was still performed in 29 per cent of the youngest age group listed, the 25 to 34 year category. For virtually all of these HRT will be prescribed.

The outcomes of 418 hysterectomies were assessed in the second study from the Massachusetts General Hospital. For those women who had the operation because of fibroids, abnormal bleeding or pelvic pain, the outcome was frequently favourable. New problems arose in some with hot flushes (13 per cent), weight gain (12 per cent), depression (8 per cent) and lack of interest in sex (7 per cent) being recorded one year after the operation in those who were not troubled by these problems before the operation.

Hot flushes were, as you would expect, more likely in those who had had an oophorectomy (14 per cent) but still occurred in three per cent of those whose ovaries were not lost. On a more positive note, only three per cent of women still had negative feelings about themselves as women one year after the operation.

It seems that many women will continue to enter menopause as a result of a hysterectomy with loss of their ovaries. HRT will be offered and taken by a majority of these women, especially in the US. Those women who have had a hysterectomy because of uterine cancer will not be able to take HRT, and so a scientifically based alternative becomes of vital importance.

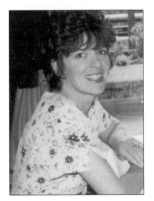

Rosanna's Story

Rosanna Haslam was 36 when she first came to see me. She owned a hair salon and had two young children. She was experiencing a whole series of unpleasant symptoms following a hysterectomy a few years before, and felt as if she had lost her grip on life.

"At the age of 21 I had to have two cysts removed from my ovaries, which resulted in my losing most of one ovary. Three years after this I had to have further surgery to have adhesions removed. In the following few years I had no further problems and had two children.

After the birth of my second child, I was 25 years old, I started to get irregular and very heavy periods. This continued for three years and I was treated with D&Cs by my gynaecologist. This procedure would help for a couple of months and then my symptoms, which also started to include extreme tiredness and irritability would return. After four cycles of this, and at the age of 30, my gynaecologist recommended a hysterectomy. After careful thought I decided to go ahead and only agreed to the operation if I was going to be left with my remaining ovary.

I recovered quickly from the operation and had no further problems until about four years later. I then started to suffer from severely sore breasts, headaches, depression, irrational mood swings and night sweats. By this time I felt really desperate, confused and frightened. I didn't feel that I could cope anymore. I visited my doctor, who was not very sympathetic and prescribed various HRT treatments, some of which helped with some symptoms like the night sweats, but generally made other symptoms worse and I felt awful.

I was getting into a worse state emotionally and becoming desperate. I found that, although many people gave me a sympathetic ear, no one really seemed to understand what I was going through. While reading a magazine, I saw an article about the WNAS. I called for advice and felt a huge sense of relief, when I found that I was talking to someone who REALLY understood how I felt and what I was going through. I made an appointment to see Maryon Stewart. I was immediately convinced that she could help me. She gave me clear instructions and direction about the dietary changes I needed to make. At the time these seemed very radical but I was driven by desperation and followed the advice to the letter. The results were almost immediate. The symptoms fell away one by one.

The following months included regular visits to Maryon and I found each time, if I followed the advice, the outcome was positive.

I have now been seeing Maryon for about 18 months. The only lapses I get are when I cheat on the diet for a prolonged period but Maryon soon puts me on the straight and narrow. I no longer use any HRT and am back to feeling full of vitality and life. I cannot express how grateful I am to Maryon and her team for the support I have had. I can now run my diet relatively easily and with my new knowledge of what works for me I can experiment with new ideas. I've been told that I look great and I certainly feel good. I've lost weight, got myself back into shape, my cravings for sweets are gone and I feel like I am back in control. An added bonus is that my libido, which was non-existent has returned completely and my husband has made it known that he is delighted to have his wife back. I really believe that all the effort I put in is worth it and I am very pleased to have been shown how to manage my menopause."

After menopause

By now you might think that a woman's hormones have left the equivalent of the Garden of Eden to enter the Wilderness. But where there is life there is hope!

Levels of oestrogen and other hormones do not dwindle away to nothing. Small but significant amounts of oestrogen are produced by the conversion of normal amounts of androgens (male sex hormones) that are still circulating in the bloodstream. These are produced by the adrenal glands, near the kidneys, and from the remaining part of the ovary. They are then converted into weak oestrogen hormones by chemical reactions in fat tissue, the skin and the adrenal glands themselves. Although low these levels are not insignificant.

Post-menopausal women who develop cancer of the lining of the womb have relatively high levels of oestrogen circulating in their body. As you can imagine, the more fat tissues you have the more of these residual oestrogens can be formed. So obesity is undoubtedly a risk factor for cancer of the uterus.

In postmenopause the levels of FSH and LH eventually lessen and with this stage comes a relatively stable hormonal situation with symptoms usually becoming fewer but with a rise in the risk of conditions such as heart disease and osteoporosis. These risks are in part due to the fall in oestrogen and in part due to age, diet and other factors but the good news is that our natural programme can positively influence both these conditions.

Confirm Your Menopause

When your periods become irregular, or if you haven't had one for a while, you might like to test to confirm that you are going through the menopause. You have two options, to ask your doctor to perform the test or to invest in a home testing kit and do it yourself.

In order to confirm that you are going through the menopause testing on two separate occasions needs to take place as a single elevated result can simply mean you are ovulating at that time. The test examines whether elevated levels of Follicle Stimulating Hormone (FSH) are present in your urine. The normal range for FSH levels before the menopause is up to 8 units per litre. When the menopause begins it becomes considerably elevated and can range up to 100 units per litre. It usually remains elevated for up to two years and once the brain has the message that the ovaries are no longer producing oestrogen, it drops back to the pre-menopausal level.

As hormone levels fluctuate during the menstrual cycle, the simple urine test needs to be performed initially and then repeated approximately two weeks later. It's a bit like performing a pregnancy test. If your FSH levels are elevated in both tests it is likely that you are going through the menopause. These new tests are now becoming more widely available. You can order the York Menopause Home Check Kit from www.beatmenopausenaturally.com or by mail on 0845 1130031.

Chapter 4

Hormone Replacement Therapy – The Nitty Gritty

For the last decade in particular the most popular treatment for the menopause has been HRT. It was pioneered initially in the US and for the first 20 years was literally 'oestrogen replacement'. It was then discovered that for women with an intact uterus there was a greatly increased risk of cancer of the lining of the uterus and so progesterone was added to make it safer. Progesterone prevents an excessive growth in the lining of the womb which can lead to cancer. Until recently HRT has been regarded as a treatment for life by many doctors. However, recent research has caused the medical fraternity to think again. It has now been formerly deemed that if HRT is the chosen treatment it should only be used for two years rather than a lifetime. In the long-term women should be weaned off their HRT and be encouraged to use an alternative approach.

HRT - The Pros And Cons

Although some women swear by HRT, they are outnumbered by the women who do not take it. Research has shown that up to two-thirds of women who try HRT come off it within the first year for a variety of reasons, including side effects or dissatisfaction. Because doctors are not widely educated about alternative treatments to HRT, women are often abandoned and left to fend for themselves.

A survey of British Doctors, also conducted by the WNAS, showed that 50 per cent of doctors said that they had problems with some women when prescribing HRT, and 43 per cent expressed some difficulty treating menopause.

HRT Risk Factors: Latest Findings

Three recent studies suggest HRT increases breast cancer risk and doesn't protect the heart. Results from the Million Women Study, published in The Lancet, show that women on some types of hormone replacement therapy may face twice the risk of developing breast cancer as those not taking it. And this increase appears to happen within two years of starting treatment and not after several years as previously believed. The greatest increase occurred in women taking combined HRT.

Two further studies, published in the New England Journal of Medicine have cast doubt on HRT's ability to prevent or treat heart disease. According to the findings of the Women's Health Initiative (WHI), women face an 81 per cent greater risk of a heart attack during the first year of HRT. A second study at the University of Southern California called the WELL-HART study revealed that HRT didn't slow the build up of fatty deposits, known as arteriosclerosis, in women who already had the condition. If you are considering HRT or already taking it you should ask your GP for advice and think about a more natural approach.

There is also an added risk of thrombosis, blood clot formation in the legs, in those on HRT. The increase in risk is two to four times and is particularly relevant to those who are very overweight, smokers or who have a previous history of thrombosis. A blood clot in the deep veins of the leg can break loose and travel to the lungs; this is called a pulmonary embolism and causes chest pain and shortness of breath.

The other dilemma for women who are considering the pros and cons of taking HRT is the increased risk of heart disease post-menopause due to reduced protection from oestrogen. Women usually think that heart disease is a condition more often suffered by men but current statistics show that 30 per cent of women will develop heart disease in postmenopause. The incidence of heart disease in postmenopause is far greater than the incidence of breast cancer on HRT, but for women breast cancer seems to be much more of an emotional concern. It was thought that HRT reduced the incidence of heart disease in postmenopause, but international studies now confirm that this is not the case, and in fact seems to increase the risk of heart disease. If you still wish to give hormone replacement therapy a try, despite the medical implications, then you need to examine the following checklist to ensure that you are a suitable candidate.

You should not usually take HRT if you have:
- A personal or very strong family history of cancer of the breast or womb
- Vaginal bleeding of uncertain cause
- Endometriosis (where the womb lining grows and subsequently bleeds outside the womb)
- A personal or strong family history of thrombosis (blood clots) especially if you are a smoker or very overweight
- Severe cardiac, liver or kidney disease
- Suffer migraine headaches
- Or have severe heart, kidney or liver disease

In exceptional circumstances it may be permissible to take HRT despite these problems if appropriate medical advice and supervision are given.

HRT may also aggravate existing conditions including:

- Moderate migraines
- Epilepsy
- High blood pressure (occasionally)
- Gall stones

HRT side effects

(Compiled from data supplied by the manufacturers of HRT preparations and from the UK doctors' guide to drug prescribing.)

Less serious

- Breast tenderness and enlargement
- Premenstrual syndrome symptoms such as mood changes
- Nausea and vomiting
- Weight gain in some women
- Breakthrough vaginal bleeding in the middle of the cycle
- Leg cramps

Minor problems

- Increase in size of pre-existing uterine fibroids
- Intolerance of contact lenses
- Certain skin reactions
- Patchy increase in skin pigmentation
- Loss of scalp hair
- Increase in body or facial hair

What You Can Do

If you decide not to take HRT, there is a great deal that you can do for yourself to help ensure a smooth passage through menopause, while at the same time protecting yourself from heart disease and osteoporosis. The basics of the successful WNAS programme are outlined for you in the second and third part of this book, together with extensive tried and tested self-help recommendations. Get a pen and paper so that you can write a programme for yourself, depending on your symptoms as you read through these sections. If you would like some help getting started or would like to be monitored through your programme then I suggest that you contact us at the WNAS to get the relevant questionnaires to complete and at the same time make an appointment for yourself. In addition to our clinics, we have a telephone consultation service that has been successfully helping women all over the world for the last 19 years.

You will find our contact details on page 112

Denise's Story

Denise Pemberton, from Michaelston-y-Fedw in Wales, was suffering with severe migraines.

"Following a very stressful period in my life when we lost three relatives in quick succession my migraine headaches reached the point of becoming constant. My doctor prescribed HRT for me as I was approaching menopause, but as it had no effect on the symptoms, after four months I contacted the WNAS for help after reading an article on their work in the South Wales Echo. I made gradual improvement during the first few weeks of following the WNAS programme and within months I felt so much better that I came off the HRT. I now only get the occasional mild headache, I've so much more energy and I'm sleeping better. Additionally, two symptoms I had suffered with for years, swollen ankles and burning eyes, had cleared up completely. I have maintained a good standard of health ever since following the programme. It's very satisfying to know that I am now in control, thanks to the WNAS."

Christine's Story

Christine was a 32-year-old mother of three from Bradford, who had a history of breast cancer. She went into an early menopause following her surgery.

"I lost both my mother and my grandmother at the age of 56 from breast cancer. My own breast cancer was diagnosed at the beginning of 1994 for which I underwent a mastectomy. Following my chemotherapy I was put on a drug called Tamoxifen designed to prevent new cancerous cells, but unfortunately one of the side effects I experienced was hot flushes. In June 1995 I was advised to have a radical hysterectomy, which involved removing my ovaries, to lower my chances of contracting other female cancers.

I was relieved to have lowered my risk of cancer, but after the operation felt very tired, with little vitality, and noticed that my hot flushes had become severe and debilitating. I knew that I was not able to take HRT because of the cancer, and therefore set about finding an alternative. I found Maryon Stewart's book on menopause in my local bookstore and decided to contact the Women's Nutritional Advisory Service for some personalised help. I had my first telephone consultation at the beginning of April 1996 and within six weeks of following the recommendations my flushes had greatly reduced and I was feeling more energetic. By August I was feeling wonderful. I was pleased to report to the WNAS that I had no remaining symptoms and that I felt I was in control of my health. My husband is amazed and has even said I'm like a new woman!"

Christine has since founded a group called Bosom Pals in her local area to help other women in a similar position. She has borrowed my slides for talks on more than one occasion.

The Weaning Process

If you have been taking HRT for some time and feel its time to make a change, it is important not to come off suddenly, for research shows that symptoms like hot flushes and night sweats can be made far worse. We specialise in weaning women off HRT over a period of a few months. First we get them established on a scientifically based alternative programme for a month or six weeks until they feel the benefit kick in, and then we suggest that, with their doctors permission, they gradually reduce the dose of HRT over a month or two until they no longer need to use it. For step by step instructions see page 74.

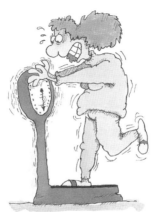

Chapter 5

Nutrition & Hormone Function

So far, we have been looking at the mechanics of menopause and how some of the symptoms in some women could be helped by oestrogen replacement. But as previously mentioned, we discovered that some of the symptoms are not particularly related to a drop in oestrogen levels, so it follows there must be some other underlying cause.

What we haven't inspected closely is our diet and lifestyle and their relationship to our health and well being, or lack of it. Our 21st-century diet is very different to that of our early ancestors.

When we examine their diet, we begin to realise that it is not 'natural' to eat meat protein, for instance, in the quantity that many of us do today. Evidence shows that the diet approximately three million years ago consisted largely of hard seeds, plant fibre, some roots and stems – a diet high in vegetable matter.

Animals today are bred to be fat. Modern meat contains considerably more fat than the wild meat our ancestors ate. Our ancestors' meat also contained more of the good polyunsaturated fats than today's meat, which is high in potentially harmful saturated fats. The ancient diet, largely composed of fresh, raw foods was also richer in vitamins and minerals.

Lifestyle is different too. As recently as the 1930s approximately four balanced meals were consumed each day, with only one or two between meal snacks, whereas now, in the 21st-century, we consume an average of one or two balanced meals per day, with approximately four or five in-between meal snacks. Convenience food and pre-prepared meals are often served instead of wholesome home cooking, largely because time is at a premium.

We no longer have the extended family to fall back on and very often women have to be the wage earner, as well as 'Hausfrau' and mother.

We also exercise far less than we used to. In the age of the car, many of us have forgotten what our legs were designed for. We drive from one place to another, do more sitting down than is good for us and allow our metabolic rate to rest!

As a result we are suffering far more from conditions that were much more rare in the past. Heart disease, cancer, diabetes and osteoporosis are just a few of the disorders that are on the increase. So too are symptoms like irritable bowel syndrome, including constipation, diarrhoea with painful gas, bloated abdomen, migraine headaches, nervous tension, irritability, insomnia, feelings of aggression and fatigue.

The Midlife Survey

In August 1999 we conducted a survey of women at midlife in order to assess their health prospects. Although we had thousands of replies, we analysed 1000 forms, 51 per cent of whom were still menstruating, and 57 per cent who said they wouldn't contemplate taking HRT during menopause.

- A staggering 73 per cent of the women included in the sample admitted to not feeling as healthy as they used to, with only 27 per cent doing adequate exercise.

- 15 per cent of the sample were smokers, with 68 per cent smoking more than ten cigarettes per day. Interestingly, the smokers were more concerned about the prospects of becoming victims of cancer than they were of heart disease and they were hardly concerned at all about osteoporosis.

- On a more positive note 93 per cent of the women said they were willing to modify their diet, 92 per cent willing to increase their exercise, and 89 per cent willing to incorporate relaxation into their timetable.

Considering that some 83 per cent had never heard of phytoestrogens, we concluded that lack of education was the underlying cause for their decreased well being. In our experience, once this is remedied long-term health prospects quickly improve.

There is now no doubt that our diet influences our hormone function. Medical researchers are beginning to work it out for women and eventually they will also work it out for men. So far it would seem that there are three main ways that our diet and nutritional state can determine our hormonal balance:

- The balance of fat and fibre in the diet

- The effects of individual essential nutrients

- The presence of natural oestrogen and progesterone compounds in foods

Before we launch into these three areas we must acknowledge that we do not actually know how important each of these components are. It is safe to say that they have been overlooked and their importance will rise perhaps to a point where dietary change will be acknowledged for some women, as a real alternative to HRT for the control of oestrogen-withdrawal symptoms. That is our impression from many of the women we have seen and advised in a clinic setting.

Fat and Fibre

This duo, who took the leading roles in the story of heart disease, have been busy at work on the rise and fall of oestrogen. Scientific interest primarily came about because of the strong relationship between dietary intake of fat and not just heart disease but also breast cancer. Those countries with a high intake of fat, especially saturated fat found predominantly in animal products, have a high rate of breast cancer. As yet we do not know whether reducing our intake of fat will reduce the rate of breast cancer. Such studies would be costly and complicated and have not yet been undertaken. What has been studied is the influence of our diet and its fat and fibre content on hormone function and thereby the possible risks of breast disease. Some of this information is relevant when trying to understand the relationship between diet and hormone changes at menopause.

In brief, the majority of studies have shown that:

- A high animal fat, low fibre diet is associated with relatively high levels of circulating oestrogen.

- Dietary fibre enhances the rate of clearance of oestrogen from the body

- In premenopausal women, changing to a low animal fat, high fibre diet can, but not always, lower the circulating oestrogen levels.

- Vegetarians and those who are not overweight tend to have higher levels of a hormone-modifying protein, sex hormone binding globulin (SHBG), in their blood. This helps smooth out the highs and lows of hormone function.

- Severe constipation is associated with a high level of oestrogen and menstrual irregularities.

- Antibiotics, by killing off friendly bacteria in the intestine, may reduce the natural recycling of oestrogen by the body.

What this jumble of information means is not fully clear. In essence, the extremes of diet and bowel function are associated with the more extreme levels of hormones, especially oestrogen. Being a lifelong high-fat, low-fibre eater, as is seen in many Western women, is more likely to be associated with menopausal symptoms of oestrogen withdrawal. This may be because their systems are used to a relatively high instance of circulating hormones and that they tolerate the drop less well. In theory, making a dramatic change to a low fat, high fibre diet might aggravate the symptoms of oestrogen withdrawal in women in perimenopause or early postmenopause. This effect is likely to be offset by the impact of improved nutrition on hormone function.

In summary, there seems to be an excess hormonal vulnerability in those consuming a Western diet. Make the change, but do not be too drastic about it at the time of menopause. For example, don't suddenly go from being a meat-eater to following a weight-loss vegan diet! Changing your diet may help not only with the risks of heart disease, but also with the risks of the hormonally related cancers in the breast and womb.

Individual Essential Nutrients

It appears that many nutrients are essential either for the production of hormones or to help the way in which the hormones do their job in the body. Nutritional deficiencies have to be severe before they have a profound influence, but several combined nutritional inadequacies will probably have a subtle adverse effect on hormone function. You may think that nutritional deficiencies are rare in countries like America, England and Australia. True, if we confine ourselves to severe deficiencies. But from authoritative government surveys, poor intake of a number of nutrients are acknowledged in a substantial number of women of childbearing age. So there is absolutely no room for nutritional complacency.

WNAS Nutritional profiles

- 50-80% of women with PMS have low red cell magnesium
- B Vitamins, Zinc, Iron + essential fatty acids were also in short supply to a significant degree

---

Let's take an individual look at some of the important nutrients.

Iron

The main function of iron is the production of the oxygen-carrying blood pigment hemoglobin. Muscles and the brain also need iron, and a lack of it causes not only anaemia but also fatigue, loss of hair and brittle, split nails. Anaemia occurs in four per cent of women of childbearing age but has to be severe to result in cessation of periods. Mild lack of iron is more likely and can be present in an additional 10 per cent of the menstruating population. It can cause fatigue and should be considered in any perimenopausal woman in whom this is a problem.

Vitamin B

There are several members of the vitamin B family. Broadly speaking, they are involved in energy release from food and the health of the nervous system. Severe deficiency of two of these vitamins is on record as causing cessation of menstruation or menstrual irregularities. These are vitamin B12 and vitamin B3. A deficiency of either of these is rare.

Lack of vitamin B12 can occur in long-standing strict vegans and in older people who lose the ability to absorb this vitamin. Weight loss, fatigue, tingling in the feet and loss of balance are other features of this deficiency.

Lack of vitamin B3 - nicotinic acid or niacinamide - should only develop in the heavy alcohol consumer, those on very poor low-protein diets and those with serious digestive problems. Depression, a red, scaly rash on the face, backs of the hands or other light-exposed areas and diarrhoea are other features. In malnourished women deficient in this vitamin, menstrual irregularities are apparently common. It might occasionally be a problem in the perimenopausal woman if she is drinking heavily.

Vitamin B6 is often linked with premenstrual syndrome. Mild deficiency, diagnosed by a low blood level, is surprisingly common and together with a lack of vitamin B1, thiamine, which is known to be common in both men and women with anxiety and depression. Deficiency of this, however, is not known to be associated with any menstrual disturbance. Vitamin B6, however, is involved in the way in which tissues respond to oestrogen and it seems to be needed by the part on the surface of the cell that interacts with oestrogen to refresh itself. Hence increased amounts of vitamin B6 may be needed by some women who are taking relatively large amounts of oestrogen, as in the oral contraceptive pill. HRT seems to have a much less disturbing effect in this respect. It is theoretically possible that the response of tissues to oestrogen would be improved by correction of a vitamin B6 deficiency.

Though severe lack of these and the other B vitamins are fairly infrequent, mild deficiency is not that uncommon even in relatively well-fed populations. Such has been the concern about the poor intake of folic acid in women of childbearing age that, since December 1992, all women in the UK who wish to become pregnant are now advised to take a daily supplement of 400 micrograms, nearly twice the average dietary intake, before conceiving. Doing so greatly reduces the chance of the mother giving birth to an infant with spina bifida. There may well be other adverse effects of mild vitamin B deficiency in women of childbearing age that are not yet documented. Menstrual disturbance is one possibility.

Vitamin E

The use of Vitamin E in women of reproductive age was stimulated by the early discovery that in rats, deficiency caused pregnant females to abort and lose their offspring. Indeed, the proper chemical name for vitamin E is tocopherol, which in Greek means childbearing. In premenstrual women, in fact women with premenstrual syndrome, supplements of vitamin E have been found to raise oestrogen levels but the response varied considerably with the dose. Its effect on hormone chemistry in perimenopausal and postmenopausal women has unfortunately not been studied. However, its effect on hot flushes has been recorded since 1949. In the earliest study a response rate of over 50 per cent was recorded when high doses, in the region of 1000 IUs per day were given.

Although the trial was not scientific enough to convince today's doctors, this early report included the case of one woman who resumed menstruation ten months after she had received radiation treatment to destroy her ovaries. So we cannot rule it out completely. Again, we would like to know if some menopausal women have a relative lack of this vitamin. Lower-than-average levels have been associated with a higher-than-average risk of breast cancer. So it might help some women, perhaps those in perimenopause rather than those who are truly postmenstrual.

We often use vitamin E as part of our programme for menopausal women: try 200 IUs initially each day.

Magnesium

This mineral has come from obscurity to the verge of fame in the last ten years. The cousin of calcium, it is necessary for normal bone, muscle and nerve function. It is also the sister of potassium and like her is found mainly inside cells controlling energy functions. Good sources of magnesium are fresh fruit and vegetables, especially green ones. From dietary assessments it appears that between 10 and 20 per cent of women of childbearing age consume less than the minimum recommended amounts of these nutrients.

Magnesium and some other minerals are also involved in hormone function.

Experiments have shown that this mineral is needed by the ovaries in order for them to respond satisfactorily to the stimulatory effect of the pituitary hormones, LH and FSH. The failure to respond to them on the part of the ovaries is exactly what happens at menopause. We don't think that lack of magnesium is the cause of menopause! However, it does often seem to be moderately lacking in women of all ages with premenstrual syndrome and we know that supplements of it can help PMS. So it wouldn't be too surprising if it was having some influence over some menopausal problems. Good candidates would include those experiencing an early menopause, erratic cycles, fatigue, depression and aches and pains.

A high-magnesium diet is very nutritious and supplements are harmless enough; the only likely side effect is diarrhoea which, for those who are constipated, might be helpful. No studies, as yet, have looked at the relationship between magnesium and either the timing or the symptoms of menopause. From our own experience we have seen a rather variable picture when we have looked at the results of red-cell magnesium levels, which are known to be low in at least 50 per cent of women with PMS as well as being low in some women with menopausal difficulties. Again, it is asking too much to blame everything on one nutrient; what is needed are large studies that look at nutritional factors in detail. We have found a magnesium and calcium supplement called Gynovite useful in treating hot flushes, and it may also encourage bone regeneration.

General dietary recommendations
Hot flushes are aggravated by:

- Caffeine (tea, coffee, chocolate and cola)
- Spicy foods
- Alcohol
- Hot drinks

Madelaine's Story

Madelaine was 35 when she had one of her ovaries removed because of a large cyst. Eleven years later, her periods were becoming irregular and even though she was not experiencing hot flushes she wondered if she might be approaching menopause. Along with her periods, of which she had had six in the preceding 12 months, she was experiencing migraine headaches, breast tenderness and lumps, and fluid retention. The breast tenderness had been partly helped by evening primrose oil.

Investigations showed significantly increased levels of the hormones FSH and LH into the 'menopausal range'. Nutritional tests showed low levels of vitamin B, magnesium and essential fatty acids of both the vegetable and fish oil types, so it was therefore possible that Madelaine's hormone function was being compromised by her nutritional state.

A change in her diet was suggested to reduce the intake of saturated animal fats and to increase her intake of the polyunsaturated essential fats. Foods known to be common triggers of migraine headaches were also to be avoided, as were salt and salty foods. Supplements of multivitamins, magnesium and evening primrose oil with fish oils were recommended to be taken for several months. These measures resulted in a reduction of her migraine headaches and a substantial lessening of her breast problems.

Zinc

This mineral is certainly important for men, as even a mild lack of it, if prolonged, can have a profound effect on sperm and testosterone production. By rights it should be important to women but we do not know of any evidence to this effect. Intakes in Australia are pretty close to the minimum recommended amounts and absorption is easily reduced by alcohol, bran and many other foods. The best dietary source is oysters followed by beef and most other meats (so you know what to give him for dinner tonight!). It would probably take a severe deficiency to upset hormone function and this is only likely in the heavy alcohol consumer and those eating a low-protein diet.

Essential fatty acids

Some fats, like vitamins and minerals, are essential. These essential fats are the polyunsaturates and monounsaturates found in most vegetable oils and oily fish. We've heard a lot about them in relation to heart disease and the story doesn't end there. They are not easy things to study. First, your body only needs a tiny amount of them, which is just as well since that's all it usually gets with our modern-day diet. A deficiency builds up over years, possibly decades, before it takes its toll. We know, so far, that severe deficiency is rare and is confined to premature infants, alcoholics (again) and the malnourished. A mild deficiency can develop in the 'normal' population and this could be a factor in heart disease. Intakes and blood levels generally fall with increasing age.

On the hormone front, essential fatty acids are doing something very interesting. These fats are used in the building of cell walls and in particular seem to influence the function of those pieces of cell machinery that are actually embedded in the cell wall, such as the receptors for hormones. So it is possible that a relative lack of these essential fatty acids over many years might modify the way in which our bodies respond to certain hormones. So what's the evidence? Well, in the cheetah a lack of the essential fishy fatty acids, particularly of the omega-3 series, results in infertility because of an inability of the female to ovulate. Sounds familiar? And in the human? Sorry, right now we don't know but again it's a possible factor. Certain specialized preparations of these essential fatty acids have already been of demonstrable benefit in a variety of diverse areas. So far we have seen evening primrose oil (the omega-6 series) benefit women with premenstrual breast tenderness and also help some adults and children with dry eczema.

The fish oils have also made their mark in reducing the pain and inflammation of rheumatoid arthritis and they help to lower elevated levels of some blood fats - not cholesterol. A number of studies suggest that combining calcium with essential fatty acids from evening primrose oil and marine fish oil may be an effective way of preventing osteoporosis. There is some evidence to suggest that it helps to increase the absorption of calcium from the diet and the uptake of calcium by the bone. We know that a lack of essential fatty acids reduces the effectiveness of vitamin D in animals, resulting in weaker bones.

Studies have established that the best combination is of evening primrose oil and marine oil as it encourages calcium absorption and reduces calcium loss in the urine. This combination contains 400 mg of pure evening primrose oil, 44 mg of marine fish oil and 100 mg of calcium. It seems that this combination may help direct calcium to sites of deposition in the bone and may thus help prevent the bone-thinning process. It is effectively the stamp on the envelope that makes delivery far more likely.

Chapter 6

Detecting Nutritional Deficiencies

Repeated government surveys show clearly that people are often short of nutrients like iron, zinc, calcium, magnesium and certain B vitamins. These nutritional deficiencies often underlie our symptoms and not only affect the way we feel, but also the way we look. If left to their own devices, these deficiencies may eventually manifest themselves as physical signs, which is our body's way of communicating all is not well, and is often reflected in the condition of our skin, nails and hair. Common problems like spots, greasy skin, cracking at the corners of the mouth, red patches at the side of the nose, pimples on the upper arms or thighs, unmanageable hair and split brittle nails all have a nutritional story to tell.

I have prepared a chart overleaf that outlines some of the deficiencies so that you can better understand the needs of your body. Have a close look; you will be amazed by how many signs there are.

Realising that you may be short of certain nutrients is the first step. The next step is putting it right. It's not just a question of taking a pill, but examining your diet and lifestyle and learning about which foods and drinks may interfere with the absorption of good nutrients.

The physical signs of vitamin and mineral deficiency

It is likely that this is the first time you will ever have come across the concept that the condition of your skin, hair and nails is directly related to your diet and lifestyle. Yes, that really means that binge eating, too much alcohol and living life in the fast lane not only affect the way you feel, but also your appearance. Be brave and take a look at the chart. Think carefully about which of the physical signs you have experienced in your life.

Lynn's Story

Lynn Carr was a 49 -year-old special needs teacher from Ireland who enrolled in our Telephone Consultation Service. She was perimenopausal and plagued by anxiety and fatigue.

" When I looked in the mirror I saw a stranger. My eyes looked blank and listless, my skin colour had changed and it looked thinner. I looked white and tired all the time and felt like I wanted to go to bed but was afraid to as I knew I would wake up and not be able to get back to sleep again.

Wrinkles: antioxidants, vitamins A, C, E, selenium,

Dry skin: vitamins A & E

Pale complexion: iron, vitamin B12, folic acid

Psoriasis: folic acid, zinc, selenium, calcium, omega-3 EFAs

Cracking at the corners of the eyes: Vitamins B2 or B6

Red greasy skin at sides of nose: vitamin B2, B6, & zinc

Cracking at corners of mouth: iron, vitamins B2, B6

Brittle nails, flattened upturned nails: iron

Generalized hair loss: iron or vitamin C

Soft bleeding spongy gums: vitamin C

Dandruff: biotin, omega-3 EFAs

Poor night vision: vitamin A or zinc

Red scaly skin rash: vitamin B3

Eczema: zinc, B vitamins, omega-6 EFAs

Red tongue tip: vitamins B2 & B6

Cracking and peeling of skin on lips: vitamin B2

Sore, smooth tongue or recurrent mouth ulcers: iron, folic acid, vitamin B12, B3

I was moody and listless and well aware that my children were staying away from me at the time of the month. I had low blood pressure and often felt dizzy and could only describe the feeling in my head as if my brain was chattering. I was constantly worried about everything and nothing.

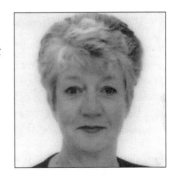

I read about the WNAS in a magazine and I immediately called them to arrange a telephone consultation. I was given a series of recommendations to follow and went about implementing them. My first follow-up appointment was six weeks later and by then all my severe symptoms had become mild. I had so much energy I couldn't believe the difference. Within another four weeks I can only describe myself as a different person."

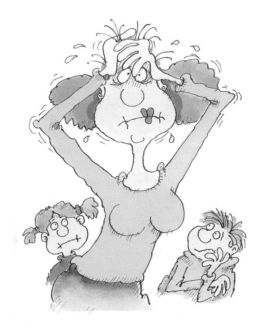

Chapter 7

Phytoestrogen – Mother Nature's Gift

What many of us don't know is that Mother Nature, in her wisdom, has given us a number of plant foods that are rich in naturally occurring phytoestrogen. These can provide us with an alternative to oestrogen if we know where to look for them. Compared to HRT, they are much weaker in their effects but can still help to control symptoms. They may also help to protect us against heart disease and the bone thinning disease, osteoporosis.

Phytoestrogens are similar in structure to the female hormone oestrogen but they are about 1/1000th as potent. Despite this, research shows that they protect us against hormonally related cancers and can block the uptake of excess oestrogen by the cells of the body.

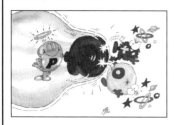

The similarity to oestrogen

Research shows that phytoestrogens protect us against hormonally related cancers, with the ability to block the uptake of excess oestrogen by the body and raise low levels.

Asian women who consume a diet that is naturally rich in a type of phytoestrogen known as soya isoflavones have lower rates of breast and ovarian cancer and fewer menopause related problems. In the Japanese language, until recently, there were no words for the term 'hot flush', largely because women in Japan, who consume a diet rich in isoflavones experience hardly any adverse symptoms at the time of menopause, unless they move away from their traditional diet.

The Power Of Phytoestrogens

A wealth of research in recent years has demonstrated that regular consumption of phytoestrogens throughout the day, particularly isoflavones, which are mainly derived from soya products, can help to control the symptoms of menopause in a similar way to HRT. Apart from being able to reduce hot flushes and other oestrogen withdrawal symptoms experienced at the time of menopause, they have been shown to have many other abilities. They may help to:

- Reduce LDL, the bad cholesterol and raise HDL the good cholesterol
- Prevent bone loss, thus protecting our bones against osteoporosis
- Maintain normal blood sugar levels (elevated in diabetes)
- Help to regulate the menstrual cycle
- Limit the growth of some cancer cells
- Boost memory powers

THE POWER OF PHYTOESTROGENS

Phytoestrogens have been shown to:

- Dramatically reduce menopausal hot flushes
- Unblock clogged arteries
- Maintain cholesterol levels within normal range
- Significantly reduce cholesterol levels
- Help to generate new bone, protecting us against osteoporosis
- Normalise blood glucose levels
- Regulate the menstrual cycle
- Help prevent oestrogen dependent cancers: breast, ovarian, prostate
- Improve cognitive function
- Restore memory

Despite this and the thousands of medical studies published on this subject carried out by conventional researchers around the world, phytoestrogens are little known outside medical and nutritional research circles. Most doctors completely underestimate the impact that dietary factors can have on our health.

How Do Isoflavones Work?

It seems that they mimic the role of oestrogen in the body and can compete against harmful environmental oestrogens, known as xenestrogens, for the receptor sites at the entrance to the cells. One of the isoflavones found in soya, known as genestein, can successfully take up occupation in breast tissue, so preventing the more potent natural oestrogen from converting normal cells into cancer cells. Because genestein is able to block the uptake of oestrogen it acts as an 'anti-oestrogen', in a similar way to the drug tamoxifen administered to breast cancer sufferers, but without the side-effects.

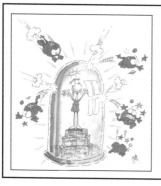

HOW DO PHYTOESTROGENS WORK?

- They mimic oestrogen's role in the body
- They compete against the potentially harmful environmental oestrogens (xeneostrogens)

Isoflavones are fast becoming known as great hormone regulators in that they can be both pro- and anti-oestrogenic, depending upon the circumstances. When oestrogen is in oversupply in the body, as can occur prior to menopause, isoflavones play 'musical chairs' with oestrogen in competition for the receptor sites within the cells.

Some of the isoflavones will inevitably displace oestrogen, and because they are many times weaker in their effect, they reduce the cancer-promoting effects of the hormone. Isoflavones also dilute the effects of environmental oestrogens (xenestrogens), which can be even more harmful to the body than normal oestrogen.

On the other hand, if you are producing too little oestrogen, for example at the time of menopause and beyond, isoflavones can give levels a natural boost, which helps to combat symptoms such as hot flushes and night sweats as well as help to prevent heart disease, osteoporosis and memory loss in the longer term.

What The Research Shows

I first encountered naturally occurring oestrogen in 1990 when I came across some research in the British Medical Journal that had been conducted by a group of Australian doctors. They had put a group of women, going through menopause and not taking HRT, on a diet rich in soya products, organic flaxseeds and a herb called red clover, all of which are rich sources of phytoestrogen. They demonstrated that it was possible to bring about the same changes in the lining of the vaginal wall in these women, as experienced by women taking HRT. This was great news for the 'alternative' camp, proving that phytoestrogens, including soya isoflavones, can reach the parts reached by HRT.

A validation of the power of isoflavones was subsequently published in the Lancet in 1992. The study concluded that Japanese women do not seem to get hot flushes and other menopausal symptoms because the Japanese diet contains foods rich in isoflavones, such as soya products.

A few years ago, another Australian study, this time of menopausal women who consumed bread rich in both soya and flaxseeds showed a 40 per cent reduction in hot flushes and a small increase in bone mass.

These studies, together with a whole host of others, indicate that phytoestrogens may well be as powerful as HRT in protecting us against both osteoporosis, heart disease and unwanted symptoms of menopause.

MENOPAUSE STUDIES

- **Manchester, England** – 60mg of soya protein for two months reduced hot flushes by half and remaining flushes were 30 per cent less severe.

- **Italian Study** – 60mg of soya protein isolate reduced hot flushes by 45 per cent in 12 weeks, and 33 per cent reduction in remaining flushes.

- **Prof Burke,** Bowman Gray School of Medicine, North Carolina, - 43 American women on 20mg soya for six weeks had marked reduction in symptoms.

- **Australian Study**, Monash, Melbourne – using soya and flaxseed bread (4 slices per day) experienced a 40 per cent reduction in hot flushes and a small increase in bone mass after 12 weeks.

Incorporating phytoestrogen into your daily diet

The richest sources of isoflavones are soya products, particularly soya milk, tofu and soya flour. Foods providing smaller quantities of phytoestrogens include organic flaxseeds, lentils, chick peas, mung beans, sunflower, pumpkin and sesame seeds, other beans, green and yellow vegetables to some extent and the plant, red clover. The problem with phytoestrogen rich food is that unlike supplements it does not contain standardised amounts of isoflavones, which can make it hard to know whether you are getting sufficient amounts throughout the day.

Foods rich in phytoestrogens are now finding their way onto the market and there are many delicious treats you can whip up for yourself in a matter of minutes. Soya yogurts are widely available, as are milkshakes, which make a handy between meal snack. You will also find the recipes for a delicious fruit loaf made with soya and flaxseeds, smoothies, whipped deserts, pancakes and snack bars at the end of this book, all designed not only to make soya palatable, but also enjoyable.

Ann's Story

Ann Higgins is a lecturer from Gloucestershire who was finding it extremely difficult to cope with life because of her constant hot flushes.

"I had the most horrendous hot flushes, night and day, which ruined my last term as a full time lecturer and wrecked my life - I am not exaggerating. I had up to 12 hot flushes and sweats during the night and felt awful as the months went on. I probably had twice as many hot flushes and sweats during the day and sweat would literally run down my face - I had to constantly wash or shower and change my clothes and felt completely debilitated and lost confidence, as I never knew when a sweat would come upon me. Within a week of starting the WNAS programme my energy levels returned and so did my general sense of well-being, and within a few short months of following the recommended diet including eating soya products, taking the recommended supplements and doing my exercise and relaxation, the flushes were non-existent and miraculously I felt like I was back to my old self again."

Try to eat the following foods daily:

You will need to try to consume 100mg of phytoestrogen in total each day in order to alleviate the symptoms of menopause. There are also some phytoestrogen-rich recipes and menus for you to follow in the recipe section of this book.

Published research, as well as our own experience, points to the fact that a daily intake of phytoestrogen is necessary, preferably in split doses. In other words they should be consumed in small quantities and often, as these compounds leave the body fairly rapidly. It is thought that isoflavones reach a peak in our blood within approximately six to eight hours. We have certainly found that by consuming a phytoestrogen-rich breakfast perhaps the phyto muesli outlined in the recipe section, together with some soya milk, and having a couple of additional 'phyto fixes' (i.e. soya and fruit smoothie or a slice of soya fruit loaf) perhaps in the afternoon and evening, you can substantially increase control over menopausal hot flushes.

ISOFLAVONE CONTENT OF FOOD Approximate phytoestrogen		content
8 oz (250 ml) glass of soya milk	=	20mg
Phyto Muesli with soya milk + Flaxseeds	=	30mg
1 Ramekin of whipped soya dessert	=	20mg
Soya fruit shake	=	20mg
Slice of soya and flaxseed loaf	=	10mg
Soya yoghurt	=	10mg
3 1/2 oz (100gms) serving of tofu	=	25mg
1 Slice Burgen Bread	=	11mg

How does this affect the daily diet?

There is no need to be put off by the prospect of introducing phytoestrogen-rich foods, including isoflavones, into your diet. There are so many different varieties that you will certainly find at least some of them enjoyable. It is not necessary to make radical changes to your diet, or to suddenly become a vegetarian, unless you really want to. If you are aiming to overcome severe and debilitating symptoms at the time of menopause it is likely, in our experience, that you will need to consume at least 100 mg of isoflavone per day initially, and to combine it with the other important aspects of the WNAS

FACT

Average daily consumption by Japanese of isoflavones is between 50 and100mg. Our current daily consumption of isoflavones is 30mg and falling.

---

programme. This will enable you to emulate the Japanese in their consumption of daily phytoestrogen, but in a Western way.

You will see from the following list of foods and drinks, with their isoflavone content, that it is not too difficult to get your optimum daily intake, especially if you also take an isoflavone-rich supplement initially which will deliver between 25 and 50 mgs of isoflavones each day. For more details about these supplements see Chapter 12 – The Benefits of Supplements.

CAN WE OVERDOSE ON PHYTOESTROGEN?

- Studies have used up to 160mg of isoflavones daily for three months and recorded positive effects

- The traditional Asian diet delivers between 50 and 100mg of isoflavones per day which seems a safe dose

- The WNAS recommend a diet that delivers between 50-100mg of isoflavones per day

---

Asian communities have been consuming substantial amounts of phytoestrogen rich food for hundreds of years with no documented ill effects. Although studies have used up to 160 mg of isoflavones daily for three months and recorded positive effects, the long-term effect of high doses has not been studied. As the traditional Asian diet delivers between 50 and 100 mg of isoflavones per day, it would seem reasonable not to exceed this dose. This matches the level that has been found to have a therapeutic effect in several clinical trials and therefore seems a good compromise.

FACT OR FICTION?

Fact 1:   For thousands of years people in Asia have eaten a diet rich in soya

Fact 2:   Asian women aged 45+ rarely experience the differences that western women suffer, i.e hot flushes, night sweats....

What about men & children?

Asian men consume between 40 and 70 mg of isoflavones daily and have done for centuries without, it seems, any adverse effects on their health. In fact, scientists believe that Asian men have a reduced death rate from both prostate cancer and heart disease as a result of their phytoestrogen consumption. Asian children also consume phytoestrogen daily, once again without any adverse health reports. Professor Kenneth Setchell, who has probably conducted more research on phytoestrogen than any other researcher in the world, believes that the earlier the exposure to phytoestrogens the better.

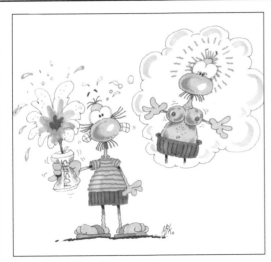

Japanese men, who consume soya products on a regular basis, have plasma levels of isoflavones more than 100 times higher than their western counterparts. This can offer immense health benefits.

- Reduced incidence of prostate cancer
- Japanese men have lower rates of heart disease

Chapter 8

Heart Protection

As you have seen, phytoestrogens have been shown to be a helpful tool when addressing the short-term symptoms of menopause. When combined with an optimum nutritional intake they have also been shown to play an important role in the prevention of a host of other conditions. These include heart disease, the bone thinning disease, osteoporosis, as well as other oestrogen dependent conditions like certain cancers, diabetes, dementia and even degenerative conditions such as arthritis.

There is now sufficient research to suggest that the majority of women can manage quite well at the time of menopause and beyond without having to resort to HRT while still maintaining a healthy heart and strong bones. This is just as well as you may remember that up to two-thirds of women who try HRT come off it within the first year due to side effects or dissatisfaction and, as you have seen, there are specific groups of women who cannot take it for medical reasons.

Heart Disease

Let us look more closely at the mechanisms of preventing both heart disease and osteoporosis.

Years ago heart disease was a rarity, and probably associated with old age. These days, in the Western world, heart disease has reached epidemic proportions, although statistics in recent years are starting to decline in countries like Australia, the USA and the UK, but they are still rising in Eastern Europe. The situation became so dire that the beginning of atherosclerosis, furring of the arteries, started to be detected in children. During the Korean War researchers performed autopsies on nearly 2,000 American soldiers in order to study war wounds. They found more than they bargained for as they discovered that three-quarters of these young men, with an average age of 22, already had the initial stages of atherosclerosis. Women over the age of 50, post-menopause, generally suffer more with high blood pressure and heart disease than men, which is thought to be attributable to the fact that they are no longer protected by natural oestrogen.

Jean's Story

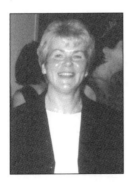

Jean Cunningham is a retired civil servant from Glasgow who, apart from any other symptoms had a history of high blood pressure and an elevated cholesterol level.

"I approached the WNAS for help with my headaches and fatigue which had become worse since taking HRT. I changed my diet as instructed, including foods that contained naturally occurring oestrogen, phytoestroen-rich supplements, and began taking regular exercise and relaxation. Even after a few weeks I had so much more energy and my friends commented on how clear my skin looked. I'd been treated for high blood pressure and both my consultant and my doctor were amazed to discover that since embarking on the WNAS programme my blood pressure had dropped into the normal range and my cholesterol level had reduced from 5.9 to 5.4."

Geography seems to make a difference

While this may sound very depressing, consider the fact that while those living in the Western World are falling like flies, the majority of Asian communities generally reach old age with healthy blood vessels. We need to examine why this is so, and we don't need to look very far. During the Second World War, when food was rationed, there was a lack of meat and dairy products. Diets were largely based on vegetarian products like grains, vegetables and beans, which meant that the consumption of animal fat was low. During this time there was also a dramatic decrease in heart disease.

Women who get menopause symptoms

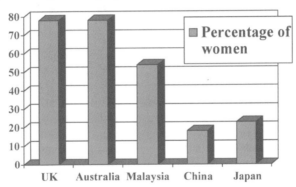

Almost 100 years ago it was discovered that animal protein, including meat, dairy products and eggs could induce atherosclerosis. In 1990 researchers at the University of California confirmed that diet can be as effective at combating atherosclerosis as either drugs or surgery. The research team used a very low fat vegetarian diet, exercise and a meditation programme on a group of individuals with severely blocked arteries, which resulted in the arteries being cleared of plaque. Other fats such as oleic acid found in olive oil and rapeseed oil, and polyunsaturated fatty acids derived from a variety of plant, fish oils and cold pressed flaxseed oil have the reverse effect. They actually shift the balance towards the good HDL cholesterol. The degree of protection that these "healthy oils" provided is under debate and of interest not only to the general public and doctors but also to farmers and politicians. Most experts in Western countries recognise a need for the 'average' consumer to reduce their total fat intake by cutting down on saturated animal fats, maintaining a modest intake of polyunsaturates and making little change to the intake of oleic acid. No doubt the debates will continue for some time to come.

Many of the known risk factors also influence the balance between the good HDL and the bad LDL cholesterol. For example, stopping smoking, correction of obesity and regular physical exercise may have a marked effect by reducing the total cholesterol and raising the ratio of good HDL to bad LDL, although doctors have not found it easy to raise HDL levels as they are largely determined by genetics. However, this is where soya and other phytoestrogens enter the picture.

The role of phytoestrogens in heart disease

It was discovered almost by accident that soya protein lowers cholesterol levels. In the late 1960s researchers set out to find out whether soya could be a palatable alternative protein to meat and in doing so they noticed a marked reduction in cholesterol levels in the soya consumers. Almost a decade later soya was again put under the microscope by Dr Sirtori at the University of Milan. He discovered that soya protein lowered cholesterol levels by an average of 14 per cent within two weeks, and by 21 per cent at the end of the three weeks. Since then, much more research has been undertaken to look at the effects of soya on cholesterol levels. An analysis of 40 published studies was undertaken by Dr Kenneth Carrol at the University of Western Ontario. His conclusion was that 34 of the studies did produce a drop in LDL cholesterol levels in particular, by 15 per cent or more. Other more recent studies have shown that as well as reducing the level of LDL, the bad cholesterol, soya has been successful in raising levels of HDL, the desirable cholesterol. Even genetically increased cholesterol levels have been seen to drop by 26 per cent in a four week Italian study, published in 1991.

Another interesting study, conducted by Dr. John Eden from Sydney, Australia, showed that menopausal women on Promensil supplements, containing 40 mg of isoflavones per tablet, showed an 18 per cent increase, on average, in the good HDL cholesterol.

A recent study by Professor Kenneth Setchell, reported at the 3rd International Symposium on 'The Role of Soya in Preventing and Treating Chronic Disease in Washington DC' confirmed that it is possible to raise HDL, the good cholesterol, while lowering LDL, the bad cholesterol. His 12-week study on 43 postmenopausal women consuming a soya rich diet containing 60-70 mg of total isoflavones each day also highlighted the anti-oxidant effects of soya.

The benefits of phytoestrogens on lowering cholesterol levels and improving heart health are an extremely important breakthrough in medicine for post-menopausal women who are no longer protected by oestrogen.

Furthermore, on October 20th 1999, the US Food and Drug Administration approved a health claim for soya protein and its role in the reduced risk of coronary heart disease and this same endorsement has recently been granted by the UK authorities. This effectively means that food products that contain a minimum of 6.25 grams of soya protein per serving will be allowed to state on the label that in conjunction with a low fat, low cholesterol diet, the product may reduce the risk of heart disease. The health claim was developed by the FDA that concluded, based on scientific evidence from more than 50 independent studies, that 25 grams of soya protein included in a daily diet, low in saturated fat and cholesterol, reduces the risk of coronary heart disease.

The Italians are so convinced about the value of soya in lowering cholesterol that it is now provided free of charge by the Italian National Health Service to those with high cholesterol levels.

GENESTEIN AND HEART ATTACKS

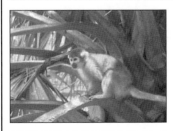

When genestein is given intravenously, vessels in monkeys dilate – restoring them to health.

There is talk of giving intravenously genstein to heart attack patients

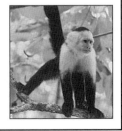

Chapter 9

Healthy Bones

During our lives, there is a constant turnover of bone. Until we reach the age of approximately 35 we lose as much old bone each year as we make new, which keeps the scales in balance. From then on we tend to lose about one per cent of our bone mass each year until we reach menopause, at which point bone loss accelerates with a further loss of two or three per cent per year for up to ten years.

In addition to the imbalance that develops between bone loss and the rate at which new bone is deposited, in cases of osteoporosis there is also a reduction in the amount of connective tissue and the mineral content of the bone. The loss of bone mass reduces its strength and increases the risk of the bone breaking if any pressure is brought on it.

As a result of osteoporosis one in three women and one in 12 men will suffer fractures of the hip, spine or wrist. Apart from the obvious pain and disability, osteoporosis often brings with it a loss of height and curvature of the spine, known as 'dowager's hump'. Within six months of sustaining a hip fracture, it is estimated that some 20 per cent of patients will die. However, what is not widely appreciated is that osteoporosis is both preventable and treatable.

Risk Factors for Osteoporosis

One of the functions of oestrogen is to help keep our bone mass at an optimum level. As our oestrogen levels automatically fall, we lose some of the protection against developing osteoporosis. This is not the only factor, however, which determines bone strength and our chances of developing a fracture in later life.

Bone density

There are a number of dietary, lifestyle and environmental factors that influence the strength and density of our bones, throughout our lives. The mineral content of a woman's bones at the time of menopause is not so much influenced by her current dietary intake but by her past intake of calcium over the previous 40 or 50 years.

Joanne's Story

Joanne Simms was a mother of two from Toronto who had been diagnosed with premature osteoporosis.

"I had a surprisingly early menopause in my early 40s and was shocked to discover through a bone density scan a seven per cent bone loss in one year and it was therefore suggested I take long-term medication for the osteoporosis. I'd never been eager to take drugs so I read Maryon Stewart's book "Beat the Menopause Without HRT" and decided to give myself a year of natural solutions before accepting the drugs. Maryon helped me to refine my programme, which consisted of making significant dietary changes, taking nutritional supplements and doing daily weight bearing exercises. The follow-up bone density scan one year later showed virtually no further bone loss so the consultant advised me to 'keep taking the tablets'. I'm hoping that next year's scan will show that I have made some new bone. I'm certainly feeling well and much fitter as a result of this new regime."

What determines the strength of our bones?

Our diet, especially our intake of naturally occurring plant oestrogen and calcium during the growing years

- Physical activity, particularly weight bearing exercise
- Hormonal factors, particularly the balance of oestrogen
- Genetic factors which determine the size of our bones and muscles
- And apparently, according to a diet and lifestyle survey we conducted in 2002 on female health writers, the age at which you began drinking alcohol. It seems women who start drinking alcohol in their mid teens have significantly reduced bone mass than is considered normal for their age.

The current diet we consume in Western countries has much to do with our risks of developing osteoporosis in the same way as it influences heart disease and cancer. Many of us consume a diet, which though adequate in the short term, does not provide a good or optimum intake of nutrients in the longer-term, thus predisposing us to diseases such as osteoporosis.

Why is oestrogen so important?

Another key role of oestrogen is to maintain bone mass and help with the constant process of bone remodelling. When oestrogen levels are optimum our bones are constantly regenerating but when levels fall calcium is no longer directed to our bones and the net result is bone loss.

Women who experience an early menopause, or who stop menstruating because of excessive dieting or exercise, will have depressed levels of oestrogen and as a result will be at greater risk of osteoporosis.

The role of phytoestrogen

Consuming a diet rich in plant foods will provide you with dozens of different types of phytochemicals that possess health-protective benefits. Apart from soya products, flaxseeds and red clover, which are rich sources of phytoestrogen, nuts, wholegrains, fruits and vegetables all contain other important compounds as well as natural antioxidants.

What conventional treatments have to offer

Calcium

Calcium is particularly important, but it may not be the only nutritional factor that has a part to play, as previously thought. Until recently calcium intake was thought to be one of the most important factors in the prevention of osteoporosis. Average intakes in the UK, for women, are around 700mg per day, the amount provided by just over 2-8oz (250ml) glasses of milk, whereas recommended daily intake is at least 1000mg per day in the UK and 1200mg per day in the USA. However, many consume less than this, and doing so during childhood and early adult life will mean that they reach middle and old age with a low bone mass and a high risk of osteoporosis.

When you examine the international statistics for osteoporosis they seem contradictory, because some of the nations with the highest calcium intake also have the highest rates of osteoporosis. Conversely, those that have low intakes of calcium have some of the lowest rates. What confuses the issue even further is that, according to anthropologists, over 10,000 years ago no humans other than infants were able to drink milk, as we lacked the enzyme required to digest lactose, milk sugar. Hence, we open the door to an alternative underlying reason for the ever-escalating casualties created by osteoporosis.

Vitamin D

Vitamin D is mainly derived from the action of sunlight on our skin and only small amounts come from the diet. It is needed to enhance the absorption of calcium from the diet.

Essential Fatty Acids

Research suggests that the essential fatty acids, EFAs, which are part of a healthy diet, also influence the balance of calcium in our bones. There are two types of essential fatty acids, the omega 3 series and the omega 6 series. The omega 3 series are derived from fish oils, oily fish including mackerel, herring, salmon and sardines as well as from some cooking oils such as rapeseed, flaxseed, soyabeans and walnut. The omega 6 series of EFAs are found in sunflower and corn oil and margarine made from them, almonds, green leafy vegetables and wholegrain cereals. These help maintain healthy skin and also influence the risk of heart disease. They also seem to help in the absorption of calcium from the diet.

Why Asians have stronger bones

Japanese women have half the hip fracture rate of women in the West, and women in countries like Hong Kong and Singapore suffer even fewer fractures. One explanation could be that Asian women are more active. Japanese women, who traditionally sit on the floor, will probably have stronger muscles and bones as a result of their regular movement, compared to a woman leading a sedentary lifestyle. But there is more to it than that, as new research is beginning to unveil.

It has been established that animal protein promotes calcium loss, but soya protein on the other hand seems to have a protective effect. Animal studies have been conducted to compare the effect of Premarin, a hormone replacement made from pregnant mares urine, and genestein, on bone health. The result showed that low-dose genestein, the plant oestrogen, was able to prevent bone loss almost as well as the Premarin. Dr John Anderson, at the University of North Carolina, who initiated the animal work, speculates that genestein's possible effects on bone may be due to its weak estrogenic properties. Bone cells, like reproductive cells, have oestrogen receptor sites.

At the time of menopause, when oestrogen levels fall, the receptor sites in bone become redundant. It is likely that phytoestrogens continue the function of the natural oestrogen that was circulating around the body prior to menopause, thus minimising bone loss.

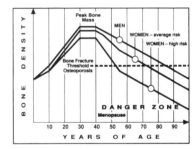

Daidzein, another type of isoflavone, also seems to be providing us with good news on the bone front. Soya products rich in both

---

PHYTOESTROGENS AND OSTEOPOROSIS

- Osteoporosis has become an epidemic in the Western world

- In Australians over 60 years of age, more than 70,000 fractures are due to osteoporosis every year

- Japanese women have half the hip fracture rate of women in the west

---

genestein and daidzein, the two main types of isoflavones, are officially approved in Europe and Japan for the treatment of osteoporosis as they appear to slow bone loss and stimulate the growth of new bone, and the same is true with red clover.

Researchers are still trying to figure out why soya seems to be calcium sparing when compared to animal protein. One theory is that as soya protein has low levels of the sulphur containing amino acids which cause the production of sulfate in the urine. Sulfate is known to work with the kidneys to prevent calcium from being reabsorbed into the bloodstream and, instead, excreted through the urine. In addition to this, most high protein foods contain phosphorus which although it reduces the amount of calcium lost in the urine, actually increases the calcium loss in our bowel movements. This may put regular meat eaters at an even greater disadvantage as meat contains low levels of calcium.

A study conducted by Professor Kenneth Setchell on 43 postmenopausal women consuming 60 – 70mg of isoflavones per day for 12 weeks, found that osteoclast activity, the bone dissolving cells, decreased significantly by 13.9 per cent and osteoblast activity, the bone forming cells, increased significantly by 10.2 per cent. These findings indicate reduced bone turnover with an isoflavone-rich diet. Another interesting study by Lee Alekel showed that 80mg of isoflavone rich isolated soya protein per day, for 24 weeks, was significantly bone sparing in the lumbar spine of perimenopausal women.

Another type of isoflavone, formononetin, has also recently been shown to help with bone regeneration. A six-month study, including 50 women, found up to a four per cent increase in bone regeneration of the cortical bone using Rimostil, the red clover product, which contains 40mg of formononetin. This rate of increase is much more than that usually seen with oestrogen drugs, which also have little or no effect on cortical bone, which is the bone involved in hip fractures.

The Way Forward

The optimum regime for better bone health has to encompass all aspects of the research. We should, of course, be including calcium into the diet, but at the same time reducing our intake of animal protein, while increasing our consumption of soya protein. It appears the calcium only crusade may have backed the wrong horse, by treating osteoporosis as a deficiency disease. If it is a deficiency, it must be of oestrogen, rather than calcium.

How can we regenerate lost bone?

- By eating a healthy well balanced diet, rich in essential nutrients especially calcium, and the essential fatty acids
- By eating a phytoestrogen-rich diet
- By exercising regularly, preferably the weight bearing variety.

OSTEOPOROSIS RESEARCH

- Animal protein promotes calcium loss, where as soya protein has a protective effect on bone mass.

- Animal studies comparing premarin to genestein for bone health showed that low-dose genestein was able to prevent bone loss almost as efficiently as premarin.

- Three animal studies at the University of Western Australia examined the role of phytoestrogens in postmenopausal bone loss. After six weeks the subjects receiving phytoestrogens had significantly reduced bone loss.

The value of exercise

At the time of menopause, when we are most at risk of bone loss, exercise becomes a vital part of our schedule, and not just a nice idea. Research has shown that weight bearing exercise, in other words anything that involves putting weight through your bones, helps to stimulate the regeneration of bone tissue by reducing calcium loss. Plenty of exercise in childhood, including sports at school, helps to build up a high peak bone mass.

The consensus from studies is that you need to exercise moderately three or four times each week, for between 30 and 45 minutes each time, so long as you do not suffer from cardiovascular disease.

Findings of the WNAS Osteoporosis Survey

We carried out an Osteoporosis Survey in the March 1999 edition of Woman and Home magazine. The survey was designed to determine whether or not there is a link between diet, lifestyle and osteoporosis. The average age of the respondents was 55.3 years and the range varied from 18 to over 80 years.

The survey shows that there is much confusion about the actual nutritional and dietary requirements for the prevention of osteoporosis in terms of the optimum calcium intake and the types of food and the quantities actually necessary each week in order to maintain healthy bones. Just under three-quarters of the sample were unaware that soya products should be incorporated into an optimum diet to prevent osteoporosis and over half of the sample were not fully aware of the importance of calcium intake in the form of dairy products. In addition, nearly two thirds of the sample were currently doing inadequate exercise to maintain their bone health.

- 5.2% of the samples were considered to be underweight - weighed less than 112 pounds.

- As many as 36.4% had at some time smoked, but only 4.4% were still smokers.

- 30.9% of the sample said that they had a sedentary lifestyle.

- Only 25% of the sample did 3 - 4 sessions of weight bearing exercise per week. 15.8% did 5-6 sessions and 11% did 7 or more.

- 9.7% of the sample had experienced one or more fractures.

- A staggering 25.6% had a relative with osteoporosis.

- In reply to the question "are you afraid of osteoporosis" the response from the whole sample revealed that 27.2% were considerably afraid, 53.7% moderately and 14.2% were not afraid at all.

- On average 50% of respondents felt that they should consume milk every day

- 11.5% felt that it was not essential to consume milk at all in order to prevent osteoporosis.

- 74% of respondents felt that soya milk and soya products were <u>not</u> important in the prevention of osteoporosis.

A more detailed account of how to prevent the diseases and conditions associated with the aging process can be found in my book entitled "The Phyto Factor" which is available at www.beatmenopausenaturally.com

Chapter 10

Boosting Memory & Brain Power

Postponing or offsetting the potential cognitive decline that occurs with increasing age must be an attractive proposition to most of us. If you have ever forgotten what you went into the room for, or lost your train of thought mid-sentence, not to mention forgetting people's names and your own telephone number, then you will welcome the prospect of help being on the horizon, especially when the help doesn't involve taking drugs or hormones.

Loss of memory is not only a problem experienced by people in old age, it is known to be hormonally related and can strike during pregnancy or after the birth of a baby while the hormones are regulating, or during menopause when hormone levels are disrupted.

The different types of memory we have are controlled by the brain. Our memory enables us to learn new things and to store millions of facts and figures in word, sound and picture form. We rely heavily on the information retained in our memory as it helps us to respond to environmental and social stimulation.

A sound memory is dependent on a healthy vascular system. When circulation to the brain is impaired individuals can experience symptoms of poor memory, lack of concentration, absentmindedness, confusion, lack of energy, tiredness, decreased physical performance, depressive mood, anxiety, dizziness, tinnitus and headache.

The brain is dependent on glucose, essential fats and phospholipids. Several of the B vitamins are essential for normal memory and mental performance. Many of the B vitamins and the minerals, zinc and magnesium, are also necessary for neuro-transmitter metabolism. Depression and alteration in mood can be associated with lack of these important chemicals. It is interesting to note that levels of many of the B vitamins in particular decline with age.

The latest survey of the elderly in the United Kingdom reveals that between 5-10% of all elderly subjects, whether living at home or living in institutions, may have an early moderate deficiency of Vitamin B12, and that an even higher percentage may suffer from deficiencies of other B vitamins.

The herb ginkgo biloba has gained recognition over the last 30 years as a brain tonic that helps to restore vascular function and memory. More than 300 hundred medical studies have now been published, most of which outline the benefits of taking a daily supplement of gingko biloba. The ginkgo extract, which comes from the maidenhair tree, increases the blood supply to the brain through the body's network of blood vessels that supply blood and oxygen to the organs. In addition, it also has an anti-clotting action, preventing the blood platelets from clumping together and thus helps to prevent thrombosis plus reducing the risk of stroke.

Ginkgo biloba has been shown to increase the blood supply to the brain and the oxygen flow to our organs. Many clinical trials have demonstrated that ginkgo helps to restore both short and long-term memory thus improving clarity of thought and powers of concentration. This is excellent news for those who, from midlife onwards, notice a decline in memory.

Vitamin E and possibly other anti-oxidants might be of importance too. They may help blood flow, including the blood flow to the brain and possibly tissue damage including that of the central nervous system. In one study where a very high dose of Vitamin E was combined with drug therapy for patients with early senile dementia an improved response was observed.

In the last few years research has also confirmed that eating soya improves human memory, and not just in the younger generation, but in groups of menopausal women. Some parts of the brain particularly involved with verbal memory are rich in oestrogen receptors, so there could be a genuine physiological link between hormonal status and brain function.

The oestrogen-like effects of isoflavones have led to speculation that soya may also help to maintain cognitive function in older women and reduce the risk of Alzheimer's disease.

Furthermore, decline in cognitive function and risk of dementia may also be minimised by a healthy diet, physical exercise, cessation of smoking and limiting alcohol consumption.

Nicola's Story

Nicola is a 46 year-old mother of two and a part-time conference organiser.

"At the age of 44, a blood test showed early menopause. I tried HRT but within days was experiencing panic attacks, depression, feeling totally out of control and suicidal. Within one week I had stopped the HRT and it took me several months to regain my composure. Apart from this, I was suffering from hot and cold flushes, night sweats, headaches, abdominal bloating, constipation, general aches and pains and continued depression.

"At my initial WNAS clinic consultation I was given recommendations with regard to my diet and supplements. I began the diet suggested, which included eating phytoestrogen rich foods. I was advised to take various supplements to boost my vitamin and mineral levels and help reduce my symptoms. After four months I am getting along very well. I feel better mentally, my memory has returned and I'm more in control and much more positive. I am relaxing now and will look into having some massage as well. My fatigue and irritability have gone, I am sleeping much better, my flushes are very infrequent and constipation is a thing of the past. While on the WNAS programme my weight has dropped to a comfortable level for me at 121 pounds without having to diet which is a delightful bonus. I am very pleased with myself and people have noticed a more rational person in their midst".

Help Yourself

Here are a few self-help tips you can implement to improve your memory and circulation.

- Reduce your intake of stimulants such as coffee, tea, chocolate and cola, alcohol and of sugar and refined foods
- Minimise your exposure to pollution and cigarettes
- Make sure your diet has a good intake of essential fatty acids from vegetable oils and oily fish
- Include soya products and golden flaxseeds into your diet on a regular basis
- Take a high dose multivitamin and mineral supplement
- Take a daily supplement of ginkgo biloba, which is used to restore memory, and enhance concentration and cognitive abilities.
- Try to exercise at least three or four times per week on a regular basis

Forgetfulness and memory loss don't have to be an inevitable part of the aging process. Consuming a wholesome nutrient dense and phytoestrogen rich diet, leading an active lifestyle, and taking scientifically proven supplements, such as ginkgo biloba, will all help you to protect and preserve your memory.

Chapter 11

Wean Yourself Off HRT

You can manage your menopause naturally and feel perfectly well without taking HRT. Before attempting to come off HRT get established on a comprehensive alternative programme. It is advisable to wait at least four to six weeks before reducing your HRT dose, by which time the benefits of the new programme will be kicking in. When you feel ready begin reducing the dose of HRT by as much as half – if you are taking a high dose pill or use a high dose patch, it is best to ask your GP to prescribe a lower dose for a month or two before attempting to come off HRT altogether.

To finally come off HRT completely the Natural Health Advisory Service recommend that:

- If you take pills either break them into two halves or take one every other day

- If you use patches cut them in half and apply one half instead of the whole patch, and wait for an additional day each time before applying a new section of patch

- If your HRT is in the form of nose spray, aim to use it less or use it on alternate days

Continue on half dose HRT approximately one month whilst at the same time following the Natural Health Advisory Service Programme closely, and then, when you feel the time is right, chose a day to stop using HRT. If you experience mild flushes during the next month or two, simply adjust the dose of isoflavones in your regime upwards until the flushes have abated and increase your intake of isoflavones rich supplements in the short-term.

The Natural Health Advisory Service Recommendations:

Diet:

Include plant oestrogen in your diet, particularly soya products incorporating soya milk with cereals or mixed with fruit as as fruit shake, tofu & silken tofu blended with fruit, golden linseeds, chick peas, lentils, mung beans, alfalfa, sunflower, pumpkin and sesame seeds and green and yellow vegetables. See page 113 for further details on phytoestrogen rich foods and page 121 for a detailed list of phytoestrogen rich products on sale in the supermarkets and health food stores.

If you are aiming to overcome severe and debilitating symptoms at the time of the menopause you will need to consume at least 100 mg of isoflavones per day initially, combined with the other important aspects of the NHAS programme which are outlined in this book. This will enable you to emulate the Japanese in their consumption of daily phytoestrogens, without making too many changes to your Western diet.

Over spicy food, hot drinks and alcohol can aggravate flushes, so let your hot drinks cool down and keep alcohol to a minimum whilst going through the menopause. Alcohol tends to knock most nutrients sideways anyway, and this is definitely a to conserve essential nutrients.

Make sure you consume a nutritious diet including plenty of foods in both calcium and magnesium such as milk, green leafy vegetables, unsalted nuts and seeds, wholegrains and bony fish like sardines or whitebait. Plus avoid fatty foods, keep refined sugar to a minimum and use Lo Salt instead of table salt to avoid bloating.

Drink plenty of liquids, preferably the equivalent of six glasses of water daily, preferably cold, as it may help to take the edge off a flush. Let hot drinks cool down and use decaffeinated varieties and herbal teas.

Keep a supply of nutritious snacks to eat between meals if you get peckish. Nuts, raisins and fresh or dried fruit are fine.

Scientifically based Supplements

At the time of the menopause we often have to put back nutrients that time and have removed. In addition we aim to restore oestrogen levels through diet and with standardised supplements initially, in order to alleviate the hot flushes and night sweats as soon as possible.

The Natural Health Advisory Service Programme recommends standardised supplements that have been through successful clinical trials.

- Gynovite is the chosen multi-vitamin and mineral supplement, for two clinical trials have shown that it influences hormone balance and bone density positively.
- One isoflavone rich supplement used as part of the NHAS programme is Novogone Redclover, which has been through several successful clinical trials around the world which have shown hot flushes and night sweats, the two

most common menopause symptoms, reducing in number as well as intensity by over 50% within 8 weeks. The other good news is that Novogen Redclover does not cause thickening of the lining of the womb, which is a complication commonly associated with Hormone Replacement Therapy. And, unlike HRT, which NHAS surveys have shown adds an average of 18lbs in excess weight in the first year, no weight gain has been seen from taking Redclover.

- There are several soya isoflavones supplements available in the market, but according to independent analysis only some are standardised and scientifically based. Phyto Soya Capsules, at standardised supplement which contains an extract on non-genetically modified soya has been found to be effective by nearly three-quarters of women who sampled it in a recent French trial.

- Another supplement that has shown to be effective in alleviating hot flushes is Kira Black Cohosh, which has been shown in clinical trials to reduce hot flushes significantly.

- Vaginal dryness often becomes a problem once of HRT. Omega 7 which is derived from the Sea Buckthorn Berry, which delivers Omega 3,6,7 and 9 fatty acids, is a new product which in a recent clinical trial has been found to enhance and regenerate the mucous membranes in the vagina.

- Other supplements that help to control hot flushes include Natural Vitamin E, Dong Quai, Sage and Ginseng.

For further details about recommended supplements see page 81.

Chapter 12

Dietry & Lifestyle Recommendations

~Based On The Successful WNAS Programme

The purpose of these recommendations is to help individuals achieve a healthy diet and lifestyle that will also help to minimise menopause related symptoms (hot flushes, night sweats, vaginal dryness and mood changes) and other menopause related health problems especially osteoporosis. These recommendations are more realistic than radical and can be followed by the majority of women whether they are taking HRT or not. More extreme dietary recommendations may be appropriate for some as part of the WNAS Menopause Programme.

- Limit Alcohol to three drinks per week or less. Alcohol aggravates flashing reactions, insomnia, and in excess can worsen or cause many nutritional deficiencies that affect our health.

- Reduce your coffee and tea consumption to a total of three decaffeinated drinks per day and use herbal alternatives. Caffeine can aggravate flashing reactions as well as anxiety and insomnia.

- Try to consume a total of five servings of fresh fruit and vegetables daily. These provide plenty of potassium and magnesium and small amounts of phytoestrogens. Where possible use organic products, or grow your own.

- Eat regularly. Aim for three meals per day as this will help to ensure a good balance to the diet and to maintain energy through the day.

- Always have a main meal that contains an adequate amount of protein from animal or vegetarian sources. Low protein diets jeopardise the balance of many nutrients including calcium, vitamin B and iron.

- Have at least one and preferably two dairy servings per day. These are milk added to cereal or in drinks, cheese and yogurt. These will provide calcium and additional amounts of protein. Low fat varieties are preferred if you need to lose weight but do not use fully skimmed milk which is devoid of vitamin A, 2% is preferable.

- Have less sugar and junk food. This includes sugar added to tea and coffee, and that in sweets, cakes, biscuits, chocolate, jam, puddings, marmalades, and soft drinks containing phosphates, ice cream and honey. Consumption of these may impede the uptake of essential nutrients and may cause water retention.

- Reduce your intake of salt, added to cooking and at the table. Also avoid salted foods like kippers and bacon. Salt causes fluid retention and induces calcium loss from the body in urine. Use potassium-rich salt substitutes and other flavourings such as garlic, onion, kelp powder, fresh herbs, sesame powder or other mild spices.

- Over-spicy food, hot drinks and alcohol and caffeine can aggravate flushes. Let your hot drinks cool down and keep alcohol to a minimum while going through menopause.

- Limit your consumption of red meat to one or two portions each week. Substitute red meat with fish, poultry, peas, beans and nuts. Dairy products, such as milk and cheese, are good sources of calcium. Use low-fat versions if you need to watch your weight. If you are lactose intolerant, go for calcium-enriched soya milk. Try to drink 500 ml (2-8oz. glasses) of milk per day, or other foods rich in calcium, like unsalted nuts, bony fish, green vegetables, cheese and cereals. Keep your consumption of all fats down to around 20-30 per cent of your total calorie intake. For most of us this means reducing fat intake by about one-quarter. Use smaller amounts of cold pressed oils such as flaxseed, safflower, sunflower, olive, sesame, rapeseed etc, and soft polyunsaturated spreads instead of hard margarines or lard. This will ensure a good intake of healthy essential fatty acids.

- Drink plenty of liquids, preferably the equivalent of at least six glasses of water daily which can include herb tea.

- Include some soya in your diet if you can. Use soya milk, preferably with added calcium, soya yogurt and other soya products that you will find on the shelves. One or two servings per day will provide good amounts of important phytoestrogens. Soya can be used as a dairy alternative.

- Include some flaxseeds in your diet, as these too are a rich source of phytoestrogens. They can be added to breakfast cereals and are particularly useful if you are constipated because they are a rich source of gentle fibre. Flaxseeds are also added to some types of bread and other grain products which can be found in our many of our supermarkets and health food stores.

- Keep a supply of nutritious snacks to eat between meals if you get hungry. Nuts, raisins and fresh or dried fruit are fine

- Consider taking some nutritional supplements to help boost your nutrient levels in the short term at least.

- Take an isoflavone rich supplement that is standardized and delivers at least 40 mgs of isoflavones each day. This will supplement your diet and help to get your hot flushes and night sweats under control more quickly. It is vitally important to ensure that the supplement you decide to take has been standardised and that the isoflavone content has been verified independently. Unfortunately, independent research has revealed that many of the isoflavone rich supplements on the market have an isoflavone content that varies considerably from that stated on the label. You will find some of the recommended supplements in our online store at **www.beatmenopausenaturally.com**

- Exercise regularly as this will produce many benefits. Reasonable targets for the prevention of osteoporosis include either walking thirty minutes five days per week and one high intensity session per week, or four high intensity exercise sessions per week and lesser amounts of walking. Weight bearing exercise helps maintain bone strength and maintaining cardiovascular fitness helps reduce the risk of heart disease, stroke, maintains muscle strength, and helps mood and sleep.

- Use relaxation techniques to control hot flushes and anxiety attacks. If severe, ten minutes relaxation in the morning and evening with slow exhalation can help significantly. Once learned, the technique can then be used at times of stress, anxiety or when flushes occur during the day.

- If you smoke, try to cut down gradually, or better still stop completely, as smoking can aggravate symptoms, especially hot flushes and night sweats. Smokers tend to have an earlier menopause. Stopping smoking at the time of menopause can reduce your risk of hip fracture by as much as 40 per cent.

Ellen's Story

Ellen Grant is a 49-year-old teacher from Sydney, with two grown-up children. She had been battling with her symptoms for a couple of years before discovering my book on menopause.

"The hot flushes and night sweats were so wearing. I got to the stage where I could hardly think straight. I know I was hit harder than some because of the ongoing stress in my life. My husband has been an alcoholic for many years, and I alone care for my sick mother, as well as teach and look after my own family. I have knowingly neglected myself, as there never seems to be any time left, which put me at a disadvantage when menopause arrived. I was so low anyway.

My friend gave me a copy of Maryon Stewart's book on menopause which I read from cover to cover. I used to take nutritional supplements randomly and have tried all sorts of other approaches to switching off the flushes, but nothing I had tried so far seemed to make much difference. After reading the book I made some changes to my diet, started exercising again which always makes me feel better and took some vitamins and minerals and one Promensil Red Clover each day. Within a few weeks, I knew that this approach was really making a difference. I persisted and managed to get my symptoms under control. The flushes and the night sweats disappeared and I felt so much better.

Once I felt better, I must admit I got a bit complacent. Life became a bit more stressful than usual, and I gradually slipped back to my old ways, and as you could have predicted the symptoms returned. It was then I realized that this highly workable programme only works if you persevere. Soon after I re-implemented the regime the symptoms were once again declining. I know for certain that this programme really works for me, but I also know I have to keep making time for myself."

Other useful self-help tips

- Aim to exercise for at least half an hour five times per week—you need to do weight-bearing exercise that is also aerobic. The benefits are a healthy heart, strong bones and a feeling of well being.

- Try to spend 15 - 20 minutes relaxing each day to keep stress levels down and hot flushes at bay. Research shows that these simple measures will reduce hot flushes by as much as 60 per cent.

- Wear several layers of thin comfortable clothing during the day so that you can peel them off should the need arise.

- Use lightweight layers of bedding so that you can adjust them according to temperature. Wear cotton nightwear instead of man-made fibres.

- Carry some cool wipes in your handbag until the flushes have abated.

- Take extra care of your hair, skin and nails: use rich hair conditioner, good moisturising lotions for your skin and nail strengtheners.

- Do toning pelvic-floor exercises once or twice a day by repeatedly holding in the vaginal muscles to the count of ten and releasing slowly.

Chapter 13

The Benefits of Supplements

Through research over the years at the WNAS we have come to realise that menopause is often the time when nutritional cracks appear. A combination of years of wear and tear, pregnancy and breast-feeding and life's stress all challenge our nutrient stores. This, coupled with a lack of knowledge about how to meet the needs of our body, results in non-optimum nutrient levels which affects our brain chemistry and the ability of our hormones to function normally.

Failure to replace what time and nature have taken away leave many women in a depleted state at the time of this important transition. Replacing nutrients including magnesium, zinc, B vitamins and essential fatty acids is vital for brain chemistry metabolism as well as normal hormone function.

Choosing Your Vitamin And Mineral Supplements

Depending on the symptoms you are currently suffering, there are several useful supplements that can be tried in conjunction with each other. The best all-round option is to take a multivitamin and mineral supplement that contains

Problem	Type of Supplement	Daily Dosage	Available From
General Symptoms of menopause	Gynovite, multi-vitamin & mineral supplement	2 – 4 per day	www.beatmenopausenaturally.com
Hot flushes & night sweats	Isoflavone rich supplements such as Novogen Red Clover or Arkopharma Phyto Soya Capsules	1 per day which will deliver between 17.5 - 40 mg of isoflavones	Pharmacy, health stores or www.beatmenopausenaturally.com
Hot flushes & night sweats	Natural vitamin E	200-400iu's	Pharmacy, health stores or www.beatmenopausenaturally.com
Hot flushes & night sweats	Kira Black Cohosh	54mg of fresh herb	Pharmacy, health stores or www.beatmenopausenaturally.com
Hot flushes & night sweats	Sage Leaf	300mg of Sage Leaf	Pharmacy, health stores or www.beatmenopausenaturally.com

Problem	Type of Supplement	Daily Dosage	Available From
Hot flushes & night sweats	Ginseng	1 – 2 600 mg capsules	Pharmacy, health stores or www.beatmenopausenaturally.com
Vaginal Dryness	Omega 7	Insert twice weekly	Pharmacy, health stores or www.beatmenopausenaturally.com
Vaginal Dryness	Phyto Soya Vaginal Gel	To be inserted twice each week	Pharmacy, health stores or www.beatmenopausenaturally.com
Decreasing Wrinkles	Arko Pharma Phyto Soya Age Minimising Cream	Apply twice daily	Pharmacy, health stores or www.beatmenopausenaturally.com
Menstrual disorders	Kira Black Cohosh	54mg of fresh herb	Pharmacy, health stores or www.beatmenopausenaturally.com
Libido & depression	Kira St John's Wort	900 mg	Pharmacy, health stores or www.beatmenopausenaturally.com
Aches & pains	Glucosamine Sulphate	400mgs 3 times per day	Pharmacy, health stores or www.beatmenopausenaturally.com
Aches & pains, osteoporosis & dry skin	Strong fish oils	1100mg concentrate	Pharmacy, health stores or www.beatmenopausenaturally.com
Osteoporosis	Rimostil	1 a day	Australian Pharmacies & www.beatmenopausenaturally.com
Osteoporosis	Calcium carbonate, gluconate or citrate	1000 mg per day	Pharmacy, health stores or www.beatmenopausenaturally.com
Insomnia	Valerian	600 mgs at night	Pharmacy, health stores or www.beatmenopausenaturally.com
Heavy periods	Magnesium amino acid chelate	2 150 mg tablets	Pharmacy, health stores or www.beatmenopausenaturally.com
Heavy periods	Iron- Ferrus Sulphate	1 200 mg tablet with fruit juice	Pharmacy, health stores or www.beatmenopausenaturally.com
Constipation	Magnesium amino acid chelate	2 – 6 150 mg tablets at night	Pharmacy, health stores or www.beatmenopausenaturally.com

good amounts of the essential nutrients mentioned. The supplement we favour which has been through a clinical trial is called Gynovite. A professor of Obstetrics and Gynaecology in the USA formulated it especially for women from menopause onwards. As well as restoring nutrient levels it is also thought to help strengthen bone mass.Once you have selected your basic supplement, you will need to add other appropriate products. Read through the chart overleaf and decide which extra supplements you need.

Laura's Story

Laura Collins is a 52 year-old Reflexologist from Surrey who has been taking Hormone Replacement Therapy for the last ten years since her hysterectomy. She felt the time had come to manage her menopause naturally.

"I gained 28 lbs. While I was on HRT and had very lumpy breasts. I was also suffering with a lack of sexual desire. I had hot flushes at night even on HRT and had developed irritable bowel syndrome.

I read about the WNAS in a magazine and made an appointment at their clinic. I felt so positive after the consultation. I gradually came off HRT over a few weeks and within six weeks the result was almost too good to be true. I followed the dietary recommendations made and religiously took the prescribed supplements. I have no flushes, I sleep better, I got my sex drive back and my vagina is no longer dry. I don't even have to rush out to urinate like I used to and my IBS has settled down. I can hardly believe I am only half way through the programme and yet feel so well".

Choosing an isoflavone rich supplement

As well as consuming a phytoestrogen rich diet, severe symptoms often respond more rapidly to a combination of food and isoflavone rich supplements. When selecting an isoflavone rich supplement it's important to choose a product that is scientifically based and has been standardized so that you can be sure that the pills contain the stated amount of isoflavones. Independent studies have shown that the actual phytoestrogen content of many supplements on the market varies greatly from that stated on the packet. For this reason we only recommend standardised products that have been through properly conducted clinical trials.

The supplement we use is made by Novogen, an Australian company, and is called Promensil. This supplement contains high concentrations of the isoflavones genestein, daidzein, formononetin and biochanin. Red clover is the richest known source of those four estrogenic isoflavones, having up to ten times the levels of the next richest source, soya. Each 500mg tablet of Promensil is designed to deliver the same dose of isoflavones as a vegetarian diet based on legumes, approximately 40mg of the four isoflavones.

It has been through several successful clinical trials around the world. One study, conducted by Tufts University School of Medicine and New York University School of Medicine, showed that menopausal women who took a single tablet of Promensil daily experienced a reduction in the intensity and number of hot flushes. Hot flushes were reduced by 56% after 8 weeks. Intensity of hot flushes also decreased by 56%, and night sweats decreased in intensity by 52%. Our own study on 100 menopausal women taking Promensil showed that 75 per cent of the sample were symptom free within four months.

Additional good news is that this particular red clover supplement does not cause thickening of the lining of the womb, which is a complication commonly associated with Hormone Replacement Therapy, and the women in the study also reported no side effects or weight gain from taking red clover.

We have now been using Promensil as part of the WNAS menopause pro-gramme for over five years and find that the hot flushes, and the night sweats, are being controlled much more quickly. Whereas it used to take us at least three or four months to control hot flushes prior to using red clover, once we included the supplement into the programme we noticed that we were able to control the hot flushes much more quickly. Patients began returning for their follow-up appointment, just one month after their initial consultation, delighted that both their flushes and night sweats were far milder.

Taking red clover in pill form is the only way you are likely to get a decent amount of it, and it is particularly good for those who don't digest soya products very well.

There are many soy isoflavones supplements on the market but they vary in quality. The better supplements are standardised and have been through clini-cal trials. As some products have been shown in independent analysis to con-tain far less isoflavones than the packet states, it is important to know which are the better supplements to try. Phyto Soya Capsules, produced by Arko Pharma, are standardised, and come in two strengths, 17.5mg and 35mg of isoflavones per capsule. They have been shown in recent clinical trials to help to reduce hot flushes and other common bothersome symptoms like insomnia, anxiety, mood problems and loss of libido.

Alleviating Vaginal Dryness

Being capable of being sexually active is an important factor for most women at the time of the menopause, but nearly half of all women of menopause age report experiencing vaginal dryness and pain during intercourse. Until recently the only two options were to either use a lubricating cream, which often didn't produce satisfying results or to use an oestrogen cream. For the last two years we have been recommending Arko Pharma Phyto Soya Vaginal Gel, which is inserted into the vagina twice a week, as it has been shown in clinical trials to actually rehydrate and restore the elasticity of the vaginal tissues within three weeks.

"I had an early menopause and to my dismay developed a very dry vagina, to the point where attempting intercourse would make me bleed. I was so sore and it was so painful that I was completely put off attempting to participate in sexual intercourse, which obviously put a strain on my relationship. Maryon suggested I tried using Arko Pharma Vaginal Gel as part of my programme. I noticed an improvement within the first month and within three months my vaginal tissues were back to normal. It's made an enormous difference and I am delighted" Kate Waters, Kings Langley

Another new product to help alleviate vaginal dryness, that has recently been through a positive trial in Denmark, is Omega 7, which is made by Pharma Nord. It is derived from Sea Buckthorn, a berry bush naturally found in Asia and Europe, which has been used in Asian traditional medicine for more than 1000 years. It is a rich source of Omega 3,6, 7 and 9 that has been shown to help maintain the health and integrity of the mucous membranes in the vagina. We began recommending that patients who have been experiencing severe vaginal dryness and even bleeding on intercourse take two capsules in the morning and two again in the evening, and are delighted to note that they are no longer experiencing vaginal problems.

"I went into an early menopause, which brought with it many symptoms including vaginal dryness and loss of libido. Sex became very painful and uncomfortable which put a strain on my marriage, as my husband is 5 years younger than I. Even within the first month of taking Omega 7 I noticed a significant improvement, my vagina was no longer dry, sex became more comfortable and therefore more regular". Jean Krane, Tring, Hertfordshire

Skin Care

By the time you reach the menopause it is likely that you will have collected a number of wisdom stripes that we commonly refer to as wrinkles. The cosmetic industry are only too aware that most of us are keen to camouflage these and reverse the ageing appearance of our skin as much as possible. There are many face and body creams to choose from and they vary in price from quite reasonable to incredibly expensive. The cream I use and recommend is the Arkopharma Age Minimising Cream, because it has been shown in clinical trials to reduce the depths of wrinkles by up to 48% within 4 weeks. It is very popular with our patients for as well as feeling good on the skin, it makes the skin feel smooth, soft and more youthful as well as only costing a fraction of the price of the creams being marketed by the cosmetic houses.

"During my menopause I noticed that the condition of my skin began to deteriorate and eventually it became abrasive to the touch and had a red appearance. It felt very uncomfortable and made me feel subconscious at a time when I was feeling far from my best because of my menopause symptoms. As Maryon was helping me to sort out my general symptoms, when I mentioned my skin problem (we had never met because I had a course of telephone consultations) she suggested I used Arko Pharma Age Minimising Cream. I used it once a day initially and it did help to some degree. Maryon then suggested I used the cream twice each day, and within a few weeks I had an absolute success on my hands. People now comment on how great my skin looks which has boosted my confidence and made me feel so much better" Sarah Adams, York

Useful Herbs

There are a number of other herbs that have a valid part to play in helping to alleviate symptoms of both perimenopause and menopause itself.

- **Vitex Agnus Castus** - shown in research to significantly relieve the symptoms of PMS, such as irritability, mood swings, headaches, breast fullness and depression. Results are usually noticeable within three cycles.

- **Kira Black Cohosh** - also known as Cimicifuga Racemosa, is a native plant of North America that contains phytoestrogens. It was used by North American Indians to treat female disorders, including menopausal symptoms.

- **Sage Leaf** - also known as Salvia Officianalis - contains estrogenic substances which can help relieve hot flushes and night sweats

- **Licorice root** - also known as Glycyrrhiza glabra, and sarsparilla root also contains phytoestrogens. They are sometimes used in conjunction with other herbs in a mixture that can be brewed into herbal tea. Licorice can cause sodium retention and increases the risk of high blood pressure in some people.

- **Panax Ginseng** - has been shown to be moderately helpful in controlling hot flushes, in our experience especially when used in conjunction with natural vitamin E.

- **Valerian** - a traditional herbal remedy for the symptomatic relief of tenseness, promoting natural sleep.

- **Kira St John's Wort** (Hypericum) - used in the treatment of depression for many years, it is thought to be more effective in the treatment of moderate depression and has fewer side-effects than conventional anti-depressants. A 12-week German study of 111 women experiencing libido problems at the time of menopause showed that 60 per cent of the women significantly regained their libido.

- **Dong Quai** - also known as Angelica Polymorphia, contains phytoestrogens, and is considered in Chinese medicine as a harmonising tonic. It has traditionally been used to treat female complaints such as heavy bleeding and premenstrual syndrome, and now has a place in the treatment of menopause sympto ms

When & How to take your supplements

Always begin taking your supplements gradually. For example, if you are due to take two or four of a particular supplement each day, begin taking one tablet each day and gradually build up to the optimum dosage over a week or two. Take them after meals unless otherwise specified. If you are taking prescribed drugs from your doctor do not reduce the dose without consent. Most of the supplements suggested are compatible with medication, and you may even feel so much better that your need for medication will reduce. If you are taking prescribed drugs check with your doctor before taking St Johns Wort.

What about the long-term?

How long you continue to take your chosen supplements is a matter of choice. Your body will usually tell you. Supplements that are being taken to address certain symptoms can be reduced gradually once the symptom in question is under control. If you reduce them too quickly and the symptoms return you can always increase the dose again. You are most at risk of bone-loss for the five years following menopause, and although the loss slows down in the following ten years, it is still pretty significant. So, if you are at risk of osteoporosis, you may well need to take supplements for some time, while having a bone density scan to check your bone mass every few years. Whether you continue to take isoflavone rich supplements will depend on the amount of isoflavones you manage to incorporate into your diet. Those who enjoy eating soya and settle into a routine will require less isoflavone rich supplements in the long term. It is advisable to continue with a phytoestrogen rich regime in the long-term in order to protect your bones, heart, memory and cognitive function.

Chapter 14

The Value of Exercise

There is no doubt that regular exercise is beneficial to us at all stages in our lives. It is, however, even more important to establish an exercise routine at the time of menopause. Not only does exercise help to improve energy levels, it may also help to overcome symptoms of depression, anxiety and insomnia, and increase confidence, self-esteem and well-being.

At the turn of the 20th century the average length of a woman's life span was approximately 50 years, and the major cause for mortality was cardiovascular heart disease [CHD]. Now, on average, women will live at least one third of their lives after menopause. These extra years that we now have are due to improvements in medication and an improved standard of living. Of course this is great news. However, the reality is that compared to our ancestors, we have become less physically active. The implementation of technology, now means that we may drive to the supermarket instead of walk, take the groceries home in the car and not carry them and employ a cleaner for the housework.

Physical activity has been recognised as being a major contributor to improved health throughout all life stages. In fact, research shows that in comparison to smoking, obesity, diabetes and a family history of cardiovascular heart disease, physical inactivity may be the prime risk factor for poor health. Furthermore, an active lifestyle has been found to improve health related quality of life throughout both women's and men's lives.

It is acknowledged that women's bodies respond positively to physical activity. They experience both improved fitness and performance. It is well documented, through research, that women do benefit from physical activity both physiologically and psychologically, so my aim in this chapter is to inform you of the health improvements that can be obtained through active living.

Weight-bearing exercise — in other words, anything that involves putting weight through your bones, so being on your feet, jogging, brisk walking, playing racket sports, weight-lifting, doing a workout, skipping or even squeezing tennis balls! - is particularly important at the time of menopause. It stimulates the regeneration of bone tissue, reduces calcium loss and thus helps to strengthen bones and prevent osteoporosis, while at the same time protecting us against heart disease.

Several studies have been conducted on groups of women entering menopause and beyond. The general consensus is that you need to exercise moderately four or five times each week, for between thirty to 60 minutes each time, so long as you do not suffer with cardiovascular disease. The pay-off is that within twelve weeks you should be more energetic, coping with stress more effectively, sleeping better, fighting off infections more successfully and feeling a lot better in general.

One study showed that when premenopausal women, with an average age of 41, trained for nine weeks, their volume of oxygen-intake improved by over 12 per cent and the postmenopausal group had an even greater improvement of 19 per cent.

Another study demonstrated that as a result of vigorous physical activity, muscle spasm was reduced and there was a significant decrease in the state of anxiety. It also demonstrated that exercising two hours before bedtime could lessen the symptoms of insomnia.

Similarly, a study of a 12-week walking and jogging programme found the women felt better, enjoyed social functions more, participated in more activities and were not so tired at the end of the day. A more recent study in the community of Linkoping, Norway showed that during menopause, very few of the physically active women suffered with severe hot flushes - in fact only six regarded their symptoms as severe, compared to 25 per cent of the less active group.

Exercise has also been shown to be better at improving the symptoms of depression and anxiety than psychotherapy. After a 12-week aerobic programme, the exercise group had fewer symptoms than the psychotherapy group and at the follow-up, one year later, this was still the case. The added bonus for the exercisers, apart from the fact that they felt much better, was that they did not have to pay the psychotherapist's bill or for prescriptions for antidepressants!

The good news is that exercise may even offset aging of the central nervous system, as well as being cardio-protective. People who exercise regularly are consistently more alert and have a faster reaction time. It has also been shown that the greater the degree of fitness, the more functionally competent the individual. Recent studies have once again confirmed that as the physical fitness of women improves, their risk of death from cardiovascular disease and cancer decreases.

One researcher, Spiriduso, concluded that "Exercise seems to be one way for people to achieve maximal plasticity in aging, approximating full vigour and consistency of performance until life's end". So there is absolutely no excuse why you shouldn't start today, unless you are currently seeing your doctor for some other serious illness.

If you really dislike exercise you are probably groaning by now. But I assure you that you will reap the benefits of your labour. We have seen so many patients who have never previously exercised begin their exercise programme reluctantly and eventually come to love it. Apart from anything else, exercise improves your circulation. Your skin will look better after exercising and you will feel more alive.

The aim is to start a gentle exercise programme to get you fit for life — you are not expected to run a marathon. It is not a competition: you are merely competing with yourself and aiming to improve your fitness level gradually over a period of months. So put the music on and start dancing! Don't forget to check with your doctor first if you have any concerns about exercising.

Why exercise?

Perhaps the most important consideration is that it is never too late to start an exercise programme. However, unlike money in the bank, which accrues interest over the years, exercise behaviour needs to be maintained if the benefits are to continue. Imagine a new drug coming on to the market offering increased mental alertness, greater energy and vitality, the ability to perform daily tasks without getting breathless or tired, greater ease of movement, faster reaction times, greater resistance to minor ailments and stronger bones. There is no doubt that the shops would be inundated and demand would far outstrip supply. The good news is that this 'drug' is a reality and available to all members of society, without a prescription and at limited or no cost. Perhaps the only drawback is that, unlike a magic pill, we have to devote a little time in order to achieve these benefits, but this is surely a relatively small price to pay for even just a few of the possible improvements.

The benefits quantified

If you have reached menopause and never been an exerciser you probably think it is too late to benefit now. Nothing could be further from the truth — it's even more important to think positively after menopause.

Bone Density

Osteoporosis is defined as a disease which is characterised by low bone mass and deterioration of bone tissue which leads to bone fragility and the consequent increase in fracture risk. Of course as outlined in the chapter about osteoporosis, there are many factors that come into play in relation to risk factors and low bone density. My focus is on the effects of physical activity on bone turnover. There does not yet appear to be evidence to show that physical activity can actually prevent osteoporosis, however, many studies have found that significant associations exist between physical activity and increased bone mass in postmenopausal women. Knowing that we are able to improve bone status is extremely encouraging. One common predictor for Bone Mass Density (BMD) during the menopausal years is whether peak bone mass was reached during earlier life (up to late 20's). Of course this information is often unknown as it is unlikely that in a fall a bone density scan would have been performed during our teens and 20's. However, identifying our activity levels during these earlier years may give a very rough guide to levels of peak bone mass.

In order to improve BMD as well as following the dietary recommendations suggested, participation in the correct type of activities is obviously of great importance as it is widely acknowledged that weight bearing activities are the key to strong bones. As you may recall from the chapter on osteoporosis, until we reach our peak bone mass new bone cells are laid down [bone formation] in abundance and old bone cells die [bone resorption] at a slower rate. However, after we have reached peak bone mass this process reverses itself meaning that the old cells will die more rapidly and bone formation becomes the slower process.

While participating in weight bearing activities an electrical charge is stimulated that encourages a transaction between muscle and bone to promote calcium deposition from the blood to the bone and to promote bone formation. In addition, it may be that in premenopausal women there is a significant relationship between increased muscle strength and greater BMD.

One further point that must be addressed here is fracture due to falling, particularly for women in the menopause transition and beyond who may have low BMD and osteoporosis. The psychological effects of a fall may be highly devastating and in many cases the recovery from a fracture due to a fall may be traumatic. Strong muscles, good balance and sensory awareness are vital to prevent falls from happening, as so often the actual recovery from fracture can be more traumatic than the osteoporosis itself. Certain exercises have been found to be great for improving coordination and balance and to actually decrease the risk of fracture due to falling, these include alternate forward lunges and travelling side squats.

Bone-Building Exercises

To prevent bone thinning, a combination of strength and aerobic activities should be included in an exercise programme. The aerobic activities should include weight-bearing activities as these have been shown to produce better results than non-weight-bearing activities such as swimming. Ideally, these should be undertaken for thirty minutes or more every other day. However, when starting an activity programme, both the duration and the intensity of the activity should be reduced. For example, ten to fifteen minutes of moderate exercise two to three times a week would be an appropriate starting-point. Strengthening exercises will place a greater loading on the bones and it is possible to target key sites, such as the upper spine, wrists, hip and ankles, which are so vulnerable to fractures. This sort of programme can take place in a gym with weight-training equipment but it can easily be developed round home-based exercises.

Upper Spine

1 When lying in bed or on the floor, flat on your back, press your head back into the pillow or the floor and push for a count of five. Release and repeat. Make sure that you do not hold your breath (counting out loud might help) as this might make your blood pressure rise.

2 Lie on your front (preferably on a hard surface) and squeeze your shoulder blades together. Then try to lift your head and shoulders a few inches off the floor. Lower and repeat a few times, gradually increasing the number of repetitions. Make sure that you don't tip your head back. Keep looking at the floor all the time so that your spine remains in a straight line.

3 In a sitting position, pull your shoulder-blades together and hold briefly before repeating a number of times.

Wrist

Stand about two feet or more from a wall, hands at shoulder height flat on the wall, arms straight. Slowly allow your elbows to bend, thereby bringing your face and chest closer to the wall. To complete the movement, simply extend your elbows smoothly and repeat. As you become more proficient, you can perform this exercise on the floor on your hands and knees. In this position, you should gradually lower your body towards the floor, ensuring that your back is kept in a straight line.

Ankles

Standing upright, bracing against a chair or worktop, lift your heels off the floor. Check that your ankles do not roll outwards and keep your weight over your big toes.

Hips

Standing on one leg, take your other leg out to the side in a smooth, controlled manner. Slowly bring your legs back together again without putting any weight on the lifting leg. Repeat until your hips start feeling tired. Ensure that you stand upright throughout the movement and don't allow the supporting hip to push out to the side to compensate. This exercise can also be performed while lying on your side, this time with your upper leg travelling in a vertical plane.

Lie on your back with your knees bent and your legs positioned on the inside of two chair legs. Attempt to push your knees and legs apart (the chair legs will prevent this); hold for the count of five and then release, being careful not to hold your breath.

Cardiovascular protection

Like any other muscle in our body the heart needs to be worked in order to be strengthened. During menopause, since we are no longer protected by the effect of oestrogen, it is not unusual for increased amounts of low-density lipoprotein (LDL), the bad cholesterol, to increase the risk of CHD. The more we exercise aerobically [increasing our oxygen intake], the stronger and more efficient our heart becomes. Improvements include the ability of the heart to beat slower and to pump larger quantities of blood through with each contraction during a resting state. At the same time more oxygen is circulated through the body and exchanged into tissues and working muscles. Of course, we must remember that other factors such as nutrition, stress levels, smoking and general lifestyle behaviours do come into play. Obviously the healthier the lifestyle we adopt, the more chance we have for the effects of physical activity, performed at the correct duration and intensity, to actually help with reducing LDL, increasing high density lipoprotein (HDL), the good cholesterol, normalising weight, mediating blood pressure and subsequently helping to protect us from CHD.

There are many reasons why exercise and physical activity are vital throughout our whole lives. However with the myriad physiological and psychosocial changes that take place during menopause, the importance of physical activity cannot be over emphasised, as you will see from the list of benefits that follow:-

The effects of exercise during menopause

Exercise increases	Exercise decreases

Exercise increases

- high density lipoproteins
- oxygen transport
- aerobic capacity
- circulation
- bone mass density
- reaction time / coordination
- well-being

Exercise decreases

- low density lipoproteins
- heart disease risk
- blood pressure
- body fat percentage
- anxiety
- depressed mood
- the effects of stress

Exercise has been shown to increase the amount of high-density lipoproteins (HDL, or good cholesterol) and reduce the levels low-density lipoproteins (LDL, or bad cholesterol). It is interesting to note that lack of exercise did not originally feature as one of the three major causes of heart disease. These were thought to be smoking, high fat levels and high blood pressure. But more recent research now considers that being sedentary carries a similar risk - hence the modern slogan that "inactivity can seriously damage your health!" So what type of activity should we consider as helping to counter the risks of heart disease? Look no further than aerobic exercise. This involves rhythmic activity using large muscle groups and needs to be sustained and moderately vigorous in order to be effective. We can see, therefore, that a brisk walk cannot only build stronger bones but can also help to protect against heart disease.

Weight control

'Middle-aged spread' can be a frustrating and depressing experience and tends to provide the visual confirmation (we do not need) of the sort of changes happening around menopause. This tends to stem from the fact that as we get older, our metabolic rate slows down. This is the rate at which we burn off our food and the calories it contains. Consequently, if we do absolutely nothing different through our advancing years, we will tend to put on weight. Unfortunately, we do tend to do something different but in the wrong direction — we generally tend to become more sedentary! Lack of time and inclination are usually given as the reasons for this and the effect is predictable and almost inevitable. If we want to maintain our youthful figures, we need to consider our dietary intake and increase our level of activity. Aerobic exercise can help to increase the metabolic rate and not just when you are exercising: the effects appear to last for several hours afterwards and, therefore, regular exercise with its elevated metabolic rate can lead to possible weight loss.

Precautions

If you have not exercised for some time, it is wise to adopt a cautious approach when starting to increase your activity levels and a brief discussion with your doctor will indicate whether any form of activity would be inadvisable.

Do remember that the old adage of 'no pain no gain' is most definitely outdated and it certainly does not 'have to be hell to be healthy'. You do not have to feel exhausted at the end of your activity: rather you should experience more of a feeling of invigoration. Listen to your body. Sometimes

EXERCISE

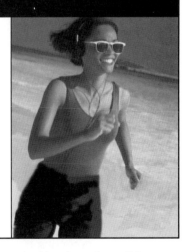

Regular exercise can help to:

- Improve energy levels
- Overcome depression & anxiety
- Increase well-being
- Stimulate regeneration of bone tissue
- Reduce the risk of osteoporosis
- Protect against cardiovascular disease
- Offset aging of the central nervous system

The WNAS recommend 30-40 minutes of weight bearing exercise 4-5 times a week (aerobics, tennis, running, skipping etc...)

you will feel you have plenty of energy, that you can tackle almost anything, whereas on other occasions you will not be able to match your previous performances. If you have a cold or a viral infection, it is advisable to skip your exercise session until you feel better and, when you resume, remember to begin gradually and not to try simply to pick up from where you left off.

If you are not used to exercise, don't be worried if you start to sweat. This is not just another one of the usual hot flushes, but an indication that your body is using more energy and needs to get rid of the excess heat you are producing. Sweating is not a sign of lack of fitness, just the reverse. The more fit you become, the more efficient your body becomes in removing excess heat. You may also start to huff and puff a little if you are working hard, but providing that you can still hold a conversation and are not in any distress this is nothing to worry about. It simply means that you need more air and that your system is adapting to provide your body with a steady supply. Gradually, if you persevere, you will find that these symptoms disappear for the same activity level and will only reappear as you begin to work harder.

Getting started

We can all think of incidents where we, or people we know, have embraced some form of activity with zealous enthusiasm, only to discover a week or two later that the novelty has worn off and a state of sedentary normality has returned. So the first rule of exercise is to choose something that you like doing. If you already like walking, whether on a treadmill or along a country lane or in the park, then do it! This is an excellent way to start. Or you may prefer to exercise with someone else or with a group of people. If so, try to make a realistic, regular commitment. This could entail attending an exercise class or going for a jog or visiting the local fitness centre or selecting a good home-exercise video, or simply singing and dancing to your favourite music. Whatever it takes and whatever your pleasure, you have already jumped the most difficult hurdle - you've started!

How long and how often?

The second rule is undoubtedly to start slowly. Many people embrace exercise with such enthusiastic vigour that they experience major discomfort and possibly even injure themselves. Deconditioned muscles being put through their paces too dramatically often suffer the consequences. This leads to a cessation of activity and the return to a sedentary lifestyle — a vicious cycle of inactivity. To avoid this common problem, 'a little and often' should be the rule. It is worth remembering that, following by-pass surgery, cardiac patients are encouraged to walk, building up to three miles a day over a period of about three months after their operation. This sort of model would be just as appropriate for many unfit people starting on an exercise programme.

Warming-up

Whatever type of activity you decide to try, warming-up should form an essential part of your session no matter how long it's going to last. It can help you to gradually get into the mood for the more demanding exercise which will follow and prepare your body systems, thus making it easier for you to perform and reducing the chances of sustaining an injury. A warm-up is designed to make you feel warm and to get the blood flowing to the muscles, so that oxygen can be provided to meet your energy requirements. This can be achieved by walking, jogging gently, marching in place, cycling or by any simple graduated activity, which uses large muscle groups in a rhythmic way. It should not be exhausting! In addition to these warm-up exercises, you should try to move the joints through their full range of movement, loosening them up and enabling them to move more freely. Joints can easily become stiff through lack of use and, by warming the fluid which 'oils' the joints, they become more pliable and this results in easier movement. Once you are warmed up and your joints are supple, gently stretch the muscles you are going to use. Try not to bounce when performing these stretches and hold them for about six to eight seconds. Adequate preparation leads to a body ready for action.

Cooling down

If you have been working hard, even on a brisk walk, your heart rate will have increased and you will often be breathing more deeply and more rapidly. This means that your heart has been stimulated to make it work harder, which is exactly what is required if you are going to improve your cardiovascular efficiency. However, just as it is better to decrease your driving speed in a car by going down through the gears, it is better to reduce your activity level gradually, rather than suddenly stopping. If the muscles don't need so much oxygen, the heart doesn't need to beat as fast, so it can gradually be allowed to return to normal. Undertaking regular activity, particularly repetitive actions such as walking or jogging, will undoubtedly lead to stronger muscles, which can keep going longer. It will also lead to shorter muscles which may be more susceptible to injury, so it is beneficial at the end of any exercise session to gently stretch out the muscles that have been working hard. Not only does this feel good but it also ensures that the range of movement around all your joints is maintained. Try also to build in some relaxation time for yourself. If you've been active, this is the reward period for all your efforts and an opportunity to release tension.

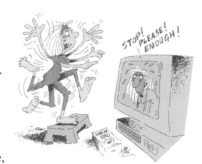

By now I hope you are convinced that some form of exercise can be beneficial, not just in helping to counteract some of the more unpleasant symptoms and effects of menopause but in promoting a healthy lifestyle, which can be maintained well into old age.

Chapter 15

The Benefits of Relaxation

It is widely acknowledged by medical research that relaxation helps to keep us de-stressed and grounded. Many women have multiple roles in life, far more so than past generations, and the resulting stress can have a profound effect on our health and well being.

Relaxation has been shown to influence hot flushes in a medical study conducted in 1984. They showed a 60 per cent reduction in the frequency of flushes in a group of women who were given relaxation training. A further study published in the European Menopause Journal in 1995 confirmed that relaxation helped to overcome hot flushes.

But relaxing may not be as easy as it sounds. When you are feeling wound up and tense, learning to release tension from tensed muscles is an acquired skill. Once you have mastered the art, however, it can be practised at any time, requires only limited space and time and is free of charge!

Instead of focusing on the outside world and the problems that it brings, you will need to learn to tune-in to your body and become sensitive to its tensions. Even if you have never been taught any basic relaxation techniques, what is involved is quite simple.

You will need to wear some loose, comfortable clothes and find a warm space where you will be uninterrupted. Either lie down on a mat, on a soft carpet or on a bed. Make sure you are comfortable with the room temperature and lighting. If you like music, you can practise this relaxation technique while calming music is playing in the background. Once you feel comfortable, do the following, step-by-step:

Learning the art of relaxation

You will need to ideally set aside at least 15 or 20 minutes each day to put your relaxation techniques into practice. Try to find a time when you can shut yourself away without any interruptions and simply lie on the floor.

1 Place a pillow under your head and relax your arms and your lower jaw.
2 Take a few slow deep breaths before you begin.
3 Then concentrate on relaxing your muscles, starting with the toes on one foot and then the other. Gradually work your way slowly up your body.

4   As you do so, first tense each group of muscles and then relax them, taking care to breathe deeply as you relax.

5   When you reach your head, and your face feels relaxed, remain in the relaxed position for about 15 minutes.

6   Gradually allow yourself to 'come to'.

Yoga

Yoga is another good form of relaxation. It has been practised throughout the world for thousands of years. It works on the principle of bringing about a harmonious balance between your mind, body and soul. It is particularly effective at helping to relieve stress and stress-related conditions. To get started, it's best to attend a yoga class and then to practise the postures at home on a regular basis.

There are many good videos which you might find helpful. From the midlife survey we carried out, we found that 19 per cent tried yoga and found it helpful.

Creative Visualisation

This is a wonderfully simple and most enjoyable method of relaxation, that requires little or no training. It is perfect for those who haven't had the time to learn how to practise yoga or meditation. We advise patients to lay flat on the floor, with a cushion beneath their head. Bend your knees and place your feet

RELAXATION

15-20 minutes of relaxation daily reduces hot flushes by an estimated 60%

Relaxation can include:

● Yoga

● Massage

● Creative visualisation

● Pilates

● Self-hypnosis

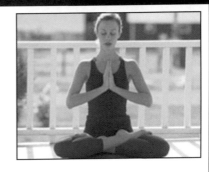

Aside from these, there are more informal relaxation techniques
– even lying down listening to your favourite music!

flat on the floor, so that you are in what is called "The Alexander lying position". Next, close your eyes, take some slow steady breaths, and consciously relax your face, finger and toes. When you feel comfortable, while still breathing slowly and steadily, you simply visualise any fantasy you fancy, from a world cruise to a good night out! The trick is to keep your mind on the trip in question. It seems to be an acquired skill, and one that you may have to work at. If you have a very busy mind, you may at first need to have a pen and paper handy, in order to download your thoughts. You need to do 15 or 20 minutes per day, and then gently come back to reality, rolling over on to your side prior to standing. Some patients feel so relaxed doing their creative visualisation, that they fall asleep!

Pilates

Pilates is one of the most recent forms of relaxation which also exercises the body at the same time. It has become very popular, particularly for people who cannot cope with high impact exercise like running and aerobics, as it offers a more gentle form, ideal for relaxation at the same time. Developed in the 1920's by the legendary physical trainer Joseph H. Pilates, the system he devised, which he named Pilates, is a combination of Western and Eastern philosophies, teaches you about breathing with movement, body mechanics, balance, co-ordination, positioning of the body, spatial awareness and strength and flexibility.

Chapter 16

Complementary Therapies

As well as dealing with symptoms on a nutritional level it is important to address any underlying problems that may well have accumulated over the years. Not meeting your nutritional needs at various stages in life, being pregnant and breast-feeding, coping with stressful situations and perhaps suffering premenstrual symptoms before your menopause, may well have left their mark. Your body may need some extra help to recover at the time of menopause, which can be provided by complementary therapies.

Herbal Medicine

Many of the herbal remedies used today were discovered by the hunter-gatherers, which gives you some idea how long herbs have been used to treat common conditions. These days many herbs have been through properly conducted clinical trials and have therefore clearly demonstrated their usefulness. As the research has been published over the years we have incorporated herbal medicine into our programme and you will find many of the herbs in question listed in Chapter 12 The Benefits of Supplements. The most tried and tested herbs to help combat the symptoms of menopause are Black Cohosh, Ginseng, St John's Wort, Vitex Agnus Castus, Sage, Dong Quai and Valerian. These all come in pill form as well as tincture which can be added to water.

Of the 24 per cent of our Midlife Survey sample who tried herbs, 80 per cent found them useful.

Acupuncture and Acupressure

Many problems that occur at the time of menopause - like hot flushes, night sweats, insomnia, depression, aches and pains, mood swings and headaches - may well respond to acupuncture or acupressure. Acupuncture will need to be administered by a qualified practitioner, and acupressure can be a useful self-help tool. Of the nine per cent of our Midlife Survey sample who tried a course of acupuncture, 74 per cent found it helpful.

Homeopathy

Where conventional medicine aims to treat people with a drug, homeopathy was developed by Samuel Hahnemann to treat like with like. The word homeopathy means "same suffering" and is designed to produce the same symptoms that you are suffering with a view to cancelling them out. The dosages are minute and often contain only an energy, or "spirit", of the original medicine. The WNAS Midlife Survey sample revealed that of the 14 per cent who tried homeopathy, 76 per cent found it helpful.

Sepia and sulphur are just two of the many remedies that may be indicated for hot flushes and night sweats. There is also a wide choice of remedies for poor memory, depression, insomnia, anxiety attacks, irritability, headaches and confusion.

Cranial osteopathy

It is worth paying a visit to a qualified cranial osteopath at the time of menopause. Not only do they provide help for long-standing back, head and neck problems, but this therapy has also been shown to reduce hot flushes. The treatment for women suffering with menopausal symptoms is often aimed at improving pituitary function, the gland found at the base of the brain, and balancing the function of the adrenal glands and the body structure.

Whichever complementary therapy you choose to explore, it is important to put yourself in the hands of an experienced and qualified practitioner. These days, all the recognized complementary specialities have official associations that keep registers of qualified practitioners. You can either contact these locally or ask for a recommendation in your local health store.

Emily's Story

Emily, a 53-year-old woman from London came to the WNAS after reading a feature in a magazine.

"I took HRT for six months but due to weight gain and general feelings of compromised health decided to look for a natural alternative. I read an article entitled 'Natural Help for the Menopause' which automatically caught my attention.

This led me to contact them and arrange an appointment to see Maryon Stewart at her clinic. The consultation lasted approximately one hour in which Maryon recommended dietary modifications and supplements including an isoflavone rich supplement to help moderate my oestrogen levels.

I was asked to cut out wheat and bran and use oats, rice and rye in place and replace cow's milk with soya milk to ensure a good isoflavone intake through my diet. After just four weeks of following the recommendations closely, my health improved and I had even lost weight!

I wasn't used to eating legumes and tofu so Maryon suggested that I read 'The Phyto Factor' which explains how you can incorporate phytoestrogens including isoflavones into your daily diet with ease. The recipe and menu section was excellent and I soon got to work in the kitchen!

When I look back at my original forms the difference in my symptoms is quite remarkable. The flushes, loss of libido and general fatigue that were severely problematic initially became practically non-existent symptoms once I had completed the programme."

Frequently Asked Questions

Q. How long does it have to be after my last period before I know I have been through menopause? I keep thinking my periods have finished, but I seem to have a period every four or five months.

A. The general consensus is that you consider that you have passed your menopause when you have stopped menstruating for one year. Menopause is actually the last day of your last period, and can only be dated with hindsight.

Q. How do I know if I am taking the correct dose of HRT?

A. If your hot flushes, night sweats and vaginal dryness are controlled adequately by HRT then you are probably receiving an effective dose. Symptoms such as breast tenderness, fluid retention and mood swings could signify that the dose is too high and your doctor may wish to reduce the strength of your medication. Younger women typically require higher doses of HRT to control their

symptoms. Occasionally blood tests may be necessary to determine dosage adjustment

Q. I have been taking HRT for the last five years and would like to stop, but I am not sure whether to stop suddenly or come off gradually?

A. It is wise to wean yourself off HRT as the research shows that coming off HRT suddenly is likely to worsen hot flushes. At the WNAS we usually establish our patients on their phytoestrogen-rich programme for the first month, then reduce the HRT by half for the second month, and phase it out altogether during the third month.

Q. I take HRT, but I have read about the importance of including phytoestrogens into the diet at the time of menopause. Is it wise to do both, or should I only do one or the other?

A. As far as we are aware, no research has been conducted to demonstrate that the two types of treatment conflict in any way. If you intend to stay on HRT and consume substantial amounts of phytoestrogen, it would be advisable to consult your doctor with a view to adjusting the dose of your HRT.

Q. Can I overdose on phytoestrogens?

A. Although in theory it is possible to overdose on many things, including water, if you stay within the range of phytoestrogens tested in clinical trials you should not suffer any adverse effects.

Q. How much phytoestrogen do I need each day to control my hot flushes?

A. The dosage used in isoflavone trials varies enormously from approximately 30 mg up to 160 mg per day. Our experience shows that it takes approximately 100 mg of isoflavones per day to control severe hot flushes. Research confirms that it is best to consume these in small quantities throughout the day, rather than in one sitting. The regular intake of phytoestrogens helps to keep the blood oestrogen levels elevated. As a rough guide, you will find approximately 20 mg of isoflavones in an 8 oz (250 ml). glass of soya milk, approximately 12 mg in a soya yogurt or dessert, 25 mg in 4 oz (100gms) of tofu, and 8 mg in a tablespoon of organic golden flaxseeds

Q. If I don't take HRT in the long-term I have heard that I will be more at risk of heart disease and osteoporosis. Is there anything I can do to protect myself?

A. HRT does help to protect against bone loss in the short-term, and it is thought that it helps to improve the bone mass by three per cent while you are taking it. However, within five years of stopping HRT your bones will have returned to how they would have been without the HRT. Although it used to be thought that HRT did protect against heart disease, more recent research has shown that this is not the case and in fact in can increase the risk of heart disease and stroke.

Incorporating phytoestrogens, the naturally occurring oestrogen-like substances, into your daily routine has been shown in a significant amount of research to protect your bones as well as your heart. It also seems to protect against memory loss. Therefore, not taking HRT is not putting you at further risk.

Q. I have read lots of articles about supplements that help with menopause symptoms like black cohosh, sage, red clover and soya products. Can you tell me, which would be the best to try, and whether any of them should be taken together?

A. Some of the supplements available for menopause are standardised, which means they are prepared to pharmaceutical standards, and they have been through clinical trials. However, not all the supplements on the market fall into this category. For this reason we have selected the most scientifically based supplements to include on our programme. We use Novogen Red Clover, which provides 40mgs of isoflavones and has been through many trials around the world. We also often use natural vitamin E, black cohosh and sage for persistent hot flushes. We also use a multi-vitamin and mineral preparation called Gynovite that is scientifically based and has been through two clinical trials.

Q. Soya products seem to be one of the richest sources of isoflavones, but I have been put off trying it because of the concerns about genetically modified soya?

A. While some people prefer to have non- genetically modified soya, from the nutritional point of view, we are not aware of any difference between GMO and non GMO versions. It seems likely that much of the research in recent years has been performed on GMO soya and varying degrees of benefit have been observed. As both varieties are now widely available and clearly labelled, it seems best to let the consumer make their own choice until there is evidence for experts to make recommendations one way or the other.

Q. Does everyone absorb isoflavones well, or is there anything I can do to improve their use in my body?

A. It seems that some people are better at absorbing isoflavones than others, and there are indeed ways of improving absorption. Both alcohol

and cigarettes tend to impede the absorption of oestrogen, and it has been well documented that a course of antibiotics can disturb absorption for several months. Reducing alcohol consumption to only small quantities, cutting smoking to a minimum, or better still stopping altogether, and taking a supplement of probiotics after a course of antibiotics will help to improve absorption.

Q. Can isoflavones be absorbed through the skin, and if so is this a way of protecting myself against menopausal symptoms?

A. Research is beginning to show that oestrogen deficiencies in the skin can be corrected by applying specific phytoestrogen rich creams. It seems that these will increase the number of new collagen cells produced, and the reproduction of new skin cells resulting in a significant reduction in wrinkles. This is good news, but skin creams do not replace HRT or the need to consume a phytoestrogen rich diet in order to control the symptoms of menopause.

Q. Should I be concerned about consuming phytoestrogens as I have been treated for breast cancer in the past?

A. As Genestein and Daidzein, two key isoflavones found in soya products, are able to block the uptake of oestrogen, in a similar way to the drug tamoxifen, which is often administered to breast cancer victims there is no need for concern. It prevents the growth of cancer cells by inhibiting the activity of oncogenes, the genes that promote cancer, and other cancer-causing enzymes. Asian diets rich in isoflavones, seem to contain a protective factor. For example, ten times more women currently die of breast cancer in England and Wales than in Korea.

Q. I tried coming off HRT a couple of years ago and developed a very dry vagina, so much so that sex became painful. I am afraid this will happen again if I stop taking HRT. Is there anything else I could do to prevent this symptom occurring?

A. Research published in 1990 in the British Medical Journal reported that a group of women taking soya products, linseeds and red clover were able to bring about the same changes in the lining of the vagina as women taking HRT. We incorporate all of these into our programme with good effect. Additionally we use two products that have been shown to help with vaginal dryness in clinical trials. One is a new Scandinavian product called Omega 7, an extract from the marine Sea Buckthorn, made by Pharmanord, which is taken daily in capsule form and the other is Phyto Soya vaginal gel, by Arkopharma, which is inserted twice a week into the vagina. The combination of making the necessary dietary changes and taking the recommended supplements are usually very satisfactory, but it takes a month or two to see a significant difference.

SAMPLE ONE WEEK PHYTO-RICH MENU

To increase your isoflavones intake at lunch time by 11mg, add 1 slice of Burgen Bread, made by Allied Bakeries.

DAY 1

BREAKFAST
Hot cereal made with soya milk
Almonds, sunflower seeds, pumpkin seeds
Chopped banana,

LUNCH
Baked potato
Pilchards
Salad with watercress, spinach and rocket

DINNER
Tofu and vegetable stir-fry
Green beans
Sweetcorn
Baked potato

DESSERT
Prune and tofu whip

SNACKS
Dried apricots
Soya yogurt

DAY 2

BREAKFAST
Soya Yogurt
Apple, chopped
Sunflower seeds, Pumpkin seeds
Pecan Nuts, chopped

LUNCH
Homemade or 'homestyle' vegetable
and lentil soup
Oatcakes or French bread
1 apple

DINNER
Soybean casserole
New potatoes
Peas, carrots

DESSERT
Ginger Fruit Salad

SNACKS
Orange
Wheat free soya and flaxseed loaf

DAY 3

BREAKFAST
Crunchy oat cereal with soya milk
Pear, chopped

LUNCH
Baked potato
Hummus
Green salad
Apple

DINNER
Roasted Mediterranean vegetables
with garlic and olive oil
Brown rice
Sweetcorn, broccoli

DESSERT
Fruit crumble with soya custard or
soya yogurt

SNACKS
Banana
Mixed unsalted nuts

DAY 4

BREAKFAST
Phyto Muesli with soya milk and
chopped fresh fruit

LUNCH
Sesame tofu with tahini mayonnaise
Tropical rice salad
Apple

DINNER
Soya mince shepherd's pie
Broccoli, carrots, sweetcorn

DESSERT
Blackberry and rhubarb compote
Soya Dream or soya yogurt

SNACKS
Pear
Rice cakes with nut butter
Sunflower seeds, pumpkin seeds

DAY 5

BREAKFAST
Banana oat pancakes
Dried apricots
Almonds, sesame seeds

LUNCH
Cauliflower soup
Oatcakes or French bread
Apple

DINNER
Tofu and sesame stir-fry
Rice noodles

DESSERT
Tofu orange almond dessert

SNACKS
Wheat free soya and flaxseed loaf

DAY 6

BREAKFAST
Banana smoothie with Phyto sprinkle
3 Ryvita with nut butter

LUNCH
Baked potato with a can of mixed beans in spicy sauce
Green salad

DINNER
Tofu sausages
Mashed potatoes
Broccoli, carrots

DESSERT
Prune and tofu whip

SNACKS
Phyto Fix bar

DAY 7

BREAKFAST
Phyto Muesli with soya milk
Pear, chopped

LUNCH
Homemade or 'homestyle' lentil soup
Soya and flaxseed enriched bread

DINNER
Salmon steak with ginger
Oven roasted vegetables with garlic, olive oil and balsamic vinegar
Brown rice

DESSERT
Soya yogurt with fresh fruit

SNACKS
Banana and date shake

RECIPE CORNER

Phyto-Muesli

Makes 10 - 12 servings
2 1/2 mug puffed rice
2 mug cornflakes
1/2 mug chopped almonds
1/2 mug pumpkin seeds
1/2 mug chopped pecan nuts
1/2 mug sesame seeds
1/2 mug pine kernels
1/3 mug organic flaxseeds
2/3 mug organic raisins
1/2 mug organic apricots, chopped

1. Mix the ingredients together and store in a sealed container.
2. Serve with chopped fresh fruit and soya yogurt or soya milk.

Note If you are constipated you will need to sprinkle an additional 1-2 tablespoons of organic flaxseeds on to your muesli each morning for the best results!

Banana Oat Pancakes

Makes 12 pancakes
50g (2oz) porridge oats
50g (2oz) soya flour
25g (2oz) rice flour
1 tbsp potassium rich baking powder
150ml (1/4 pint) unsweetened soya milk
2 bananas, thinly sliced

1. In a bowl, combine the oats, flours and baking powder. Add the soya milk, and blend well with the flour and oat mixture until a thin batter is formed. Fold in the banana slices.
2. Pour sufficient batter mixture into a

lightly oiled non-stick frying pan and cook until bubbles appear on the surface. Flip the pancake over and cook on the other side for about 1 minute.

3. Serve the pancakes warm with pure maple syrup, soya yogurt and chopped fresh fruit.

Crunchy Almond Muesli

Serves 8
450g (1lb) rolled oats
100g (4oz) sunflower seeds
225g (8oz) chopped almonds
150ml (1/4 pint) brown rice syrup
150ml (1/4 pint) soya oil
150ml (1/4 pint) unsweetened apple juice
225g (8oz) raisins, unsulphured
100g (4oz) desiccated coconut

1. Preheat the oven to 150°C/300°F/gas mark 2. Mix the oats, sunflower sees and almonds together in a large bowl.
2. Blend the syrup, oil, and apple juice together in a jug and pour over the oat and almond mixture.
3. Spread this mixture onto a making tray and bake for 35 minutes, until lightly browned, stirring every 5-10 mins.
4. Allow to cool, then stir in the raisins and coconut. Store in an airtight container and serve with soya milk or soya yogurt.

Prune and tofu dessert

Serves 4
100g (4oz) - un-sulphured prunes
200g (8oz) - tofu
2 tbsp. natural maple syrup or honey

1. Soak the prunes overnight. Drain and place in a saucepan with sufficient fresh water to cover. Simmer for 10-15 minutes until really tender.
2. Drain again (reserving the liquid) and place in a blender together with the tofu and syrup or honey, and blend thoroughly
3. Add just enough cooking liquid to make a thick but soft puree and blend. Pour into 4 sundae glasses and chill until ready to serve.

Soya and rice pancakes

Serves 4
50g (2 oz) - rice flour
50g (2 oz) - soya flour
1 small egg
250g (10 oz) - soya milk
a little soya oil

1. Make a thin batter with the flours, egg and milk.
2. Use paper towels to wipe a small non-stick frying pan with a little oil and heat until the oil is smoking.
3. Pour a generous 2 tablespoons of the batter into the pan and swirl it around to cover the bottom. Cook for 60 seconds.
4. Flip it over and cook for a further few seconds. Set aside.
5. Repeat the procedure until you have used up all the batter.

Creamy banana date shake

Serves 2
75g (3 oz) - pure apple juice
50g (2 oz) - silken tofu
1 small banana (very ripe)
4 dates

1. In a blender, combine the apple juice, tofu, banana and dates and blend until smooth.
2. Chill well before serving, adding ice cubes if desired.

Banana shake

Serves 4
4 mugs cold soya milk
4 very ripe bananas
4 tbs ground almonds
1/4 tsp ground nutmeg

1. Put all of the ingredients in a blender and blend to a thick, frothy consistency.
2. Pour into chilled glasses and serve immediately with a garnish of flaked almonds.

Rhubarb and blackberry smoothie

Serves 4
400g (1 lb) rhubarb, washed and trimmed
400g (1 lb) blackberries, washed
4 mug cold soya milk
20 ice cubes, crushed
1/4 tsp vanilla essence

1. Place all the ingredients into a blender or food processor until frothy.
2. Serve well chilled with extra ice cubes if wished.

Phyto Sprinkle

An excellent source of phytoestrogens which can be conveniently combined into your daily diet. Use in bread and cake recipes or sprinkle over your breakfast cereals, salads and desserts

1/2 mug almonds
1/2 mug sunflower seeds
1/2 mug pumpkin seeds
1/2 mug golden flaxseeds

1. Grind the ingredients together in a blender to a coarse consistency.
2. Store in a sealed container.

Wheat free soya and flaxseed loaf

Makes 12 slices
100g (4 oz) - soya flour
50g (2 oz) - potato flour
50g (2 oz) - rice flour
100g (4 oz) - Linusit Gold Golden flaxseeds (whole)
100g (4 oz) - oat bran (or rice bran if on a gluten free diet)
50g (2 oz) - sunflower seeds
200g (8 oz) - dried fruit of your choice i.e raisins or organic apricots chopped
2 pieces stem ginger (chopped very finely)
1/2 teaspoon each of: nutmeg, cinnamon and ginger
850ml (1 1/2 pints) approximately soya milk

1. Mix all dry ingredients in a large bowl.
2. Pour the soya milk over the dry ingredients and stir well.
3. Leave to stand for approximately 1 hour.
4. Spoon into 2 x 1lb or 1 x 2lb prepared loaf pans.
5. Bake at 350°F for approximately 1 1/2 hours or until firm on top.
6. Remove from pans and leave to cool on a wire rack.
7. Serve warm or cold with butter, cheese and fruit or nut spreads.

Cauliflower Soup

Serves 4
50g (2oz) soya margarine
100g (4oz) soya flour
250ml (½ pint) soya milk
900ml (1½ pints) vegetable stock
1 large cauliflower, stalk removed and broken into florets
1 tsp dried chervil
black pepper, to taste

1. Melt the margarine in a large saucepan. Add the soya flour and cook for 1 minute, stirring constantly. remove from the heat and gradually stir in the soya milk and stock until the mixture is smooth.
2. Add the cauliflower, chervil and black pepper and simmer gently for 15 minutes or until the cauliflower is just soft. Mash the cauliflower well or puree in a blender or food processor, and serve piping hot.

Hummus

Serves 4
225g (8oz) chickpeas
550ml (1 pint) water
3 lemons
5 garlic cloves
2 tbsp (30ml) tahini
150g (6oz) sesame seeds
2 tbsp soya oil
Paprika to taste

1. Soak the chick peas overnight in 550ml (1 pint) of water. Drain and wash the peas.
2. Place the chick peas in 550ml (1 pint) of fresh water and bring to the boil and simmer gently for 2 hours or until tender.
3. Drain the peas.
4. Place the sesame seeds, tahini, garlic, soya oil and half the lemon juice in a blender and reduce to a smooth puree.
5. Add the cooked chick peas a few at a time to the mixture in the blender, together with the remaining lemon juice and blend until smooth.
6. Add a small amount of paprika to produce a spicy taste if required.
7. Serve with rice cakes.

Lentil bolognaise

Serves 4
100g (4oz) - 1/2 cup brown lentils
1/2 green pepper
1 carrot
1 cup water
1tsp dried oregano
1tsp dried basil
1 onion
1 stock celery
1 clove garlic
550ml (1pt) tomato passata
1 bay leaf
black pepper to taste

1. Wash the lentils well.
2. Finely chop the onion, green pepper and celery. Dice the carrot and press the garlic cloves.
3. Place all the ingredients into a pan, bring to a boil and simmer covered, for 30 minutes or until lentils are soft but not mushy.

Tofu, herb and bean stir-fry

Serves 4
2 tablespoons soya oil
250g (10oz) - tofu, drained, dried
and cut into cubes
2 garlic cloves, crushed
300g (12oz) - green beans
3 tablespoons chopped fresh herbs
(thyme, parsley, chervil and chives)
4 spring onions, thinly sliced
2 tablespoons tamari sauce

1. Heat 1 tablespoon of the soya oil
in a frying pan or wok.
2. When the oil is hot, add the tofu
and garlic and stir-fry for 2 minutes.
Lift out with a slotted spoon and drain.
3. Heat the remaining oil in the pan
and, when hot, add the green beans
and stir-fry gently for 4-5 minutes.
4. Add the herbs, spring onion and
tamari sauce, and stir-fry for a further
minute.
5. Return the tofu to the pan and heat
thoroughly for 1 minute, then serve
immediately, with rice or noodles.

Salmon Steaks with Ginger

Serves 2
2 salmon steaks
2 tbsp lemon juice
2.5 cm (1 inch) square of fresh root
ginger, peeled and finely chopped
Black pepper, to taste

1. Place each salmon steak on a large
piece of foil. Add 1 tbsp of lemon
juice and half the chopped ginger to
each steak. Season with a little black
pepper.

2. Wrap the steaks individually in foil
to make two parcels and bake in a
preheat oven at 180°C/350°F/gas
mark 4 for 20 minutes. Serve hot
with vegetables or cold with a salad.

Ginger Fruit Salad

Serves 4-6
Juice of 2 oranges
3tbsp juice from stem ginger jar
25g (1oz) unrefined soft brown sugar
2 oranges
1 ogen melon, weighing about 1kg
(2lb)
3 dessert apple
2 pieces of preserved stem ginger,
finely chopped
fresh mint leaves, to decorate

1. Put the orange juice in a saucepan
with the stem ginger juice and sugar.
Heat gently until the sugar has dis-
solved. Bring to the boil and boil for
about 5 minutes or until syrupy.
Remove from the heat and leave to
cool.
2. Peel the oranges, removing the
pith, and slice into thick rings. Cut
the rings into quarters, removing any
pips.
3. Cut the melon in half, remove the
seeds and scoop out the flesh, using
a melon baller if possible.
4. Peel and core the apples, then
chop roughly.
5. Put all the fruit into a serving bowl,
or into the empty melon halves, with
the ginger and sugar syrup. Stir well,
cover and chill for 1-2 hours.
Decorate with mint.

Raspberry and Tofu Brulée

Serves4
275g (10oz) packet silken tofu
2 tbsp clear honey
200g (7oz) frozen raspberries
3 tbsp unrefined soft brown sugar

1. Place the tofu, honey and raspberries in a food processor or liquidiser, and blend until smooth.
2. Divide the mixture between 4 ramekin dishes.
3. Sprinkle the sugar over each dish and place under a hot grill until golden and the sugar forms a hard layer.

Phyto Fix bars

50g (2oz) - sesame seeds
100g (4oz) - golden flaxseeds
50g (2oz) - sunflower seeds
50g (2oz) - pumpkin seeds
100g (4oz) - vine fruits (sultanas, raisins, currants)
50g (2oz) - chopped dried apricots
75g (3oz) - soya protein isolate
100g (4oz) - puffed rice
100g (4 oz) - date syrup
50g (2oz) - ginger or rice syrup
2 tsp. all spice
2 tsp. ginger powder (optional)
125g (5 oz) - soya milk

1. Mix the dry ingredients together in a bowl. Add the milk and mix thoroughly
2. Grease a Swiss roll baking tray. Transfer mixture to the baking tray and smooth over the surface making sure the mixture is distributed evenly.

4. Bake at 350 F in a convection oven for 20 minutes.
5. Remove from the oven and cut into 8 equal sized strips.

PHYTO RICH FOODS

Soya beans
Chick peas
Butter beans
Black cohosh
Ginseng
Haricot beans
Hops
Lentils
Mung beans
Peas
Sunflower seeds
Pumpkin seeds
Kidney beans
Rhubarb
Sesame seeds
Red clover
Alfalfa
Split beans

Nutritional Content of Food

Unless stated otherwise, foods listed are raw.

Vitamin A – Retinol
Micrograms per 100 g (3.5 oz)

Skimmed milk	1
Semi-skimmed milk	21
Grilled herring	49
Whole milk	52
Porridge made with milk	56
Cheddar cheese	325
Margarine	800
Butter	815
Lamb's liver	15,000

Vitamin B1 – Thiamin
Milligrams per 100 g (3.5 oz)

Peaches	0.02
Cottage cheese	0.02
Cox's apple	0.03
Full-fat milk	0.04
Skimmed milk	0.04
Semi-skimmed milk	0.04
Cheddar cheese	0.04
Bananas	0.04
White grapes	0.04
French beans	0.04
Low-fat yoghurt	0.05
Cantaloupe melon	0.05
Tomato	0.06
Green peppers, raw	0.07
Boiled egg	0.08
Roast chicken	0.08
Grilled cod	0.08
Haddock, steamed	0.08
Roast turkey	0.09
Mackerel, cooked	0.09
Savoy cabbage, boiled	0.10

Oranges	0.10
Brussels sprouts	0.10
Potatoes, new, boiled	0.11
Soya beans, boiled	0.12
Red peppers, raw	0.12
Lentils, boiled	0.14
Steamed salmon	0.20
Corn	0.20
White spaghetti, boiled	0.21
Almonds	0.24
White self-raising flour	0.30
Plaice, steamed	0.30
Bacon, cooked	0.35
Walnuts	0.40
Wholemeal flour	0.47
Lamb's kidney	0.49
Brazil nuts	1.00
Cornflakes	1.00
Rice Krispies	1.00
Wheatgerm	2.01

Vitamin B2 – Riboflavin
Milligrams per 100 g (3.5 oz)

Cabbage, boiled	0.01
Potatoes, boiled	0.01
Brown rice, boiled	0.02
Pear	0.03
Wholemeal spaghetti, boiled	0.03
White self-raising flour	0.03
Orange	0.04
Spinach, boiled in salted water	0.05
Baked beans	0.06
Banana	0.06
White bread	0.06
Green peppers, raw	0.08
Lentils, boiled	0.08

Hovis	0.09
Soya beans, boiled	0.09
Wholemeal bread	0.09
Wholemeal flour	0.09
Peanuts	0.10
Baked salmon	0.11
Red peppers, raw	0.15
Full-fat milk	0.17
Avocado	0.18
Grilled herring	0.18
Semi-skimmed milk	0.18
Roast chicken	0.19
Roast turkey	0.21
Cottage cheese	0.26
Soya flour	0.31
Boiled prawns	0.34
Boiled egg	0.35
Topside of beef, cooked	0.35
Leg of lamb, cooked	0.38
Cheddar cheese	0.40
Muesli	0.70
Almonds	0.75
Cornflakes	1.50
Rice Krispies	1.50

Vitamin B3 – Niacin
Milligrams per 100 g (3.5 oz)

Boiled egg	0.07
Cheddar cheese	0.07
Full-fat milk	0.08
Skimmed milk	0.09
Semi-skimmed milk	0.09
Cottage cheese	0.13
Cox's apple	0.20
Cabbage, boiled	0.30
Orange	0.40
Baked beans	0.50
Potatoes, boiled	0.50
Soya beans, boiled	0.50
Lentils, boiled	0.60
Banana	0.70
Tomato	1.00
Avocado	1.10
Green peppers, raw	1.10
Brown rice	1.30
Wholemeal spaghetti, boiled	1.30
White self-raising flour	1.50
Grilled cod	1.70
White bread	1.70
Soya flour	2.00
Red peppers, raw	2.20

Almonds	3.10
Grilled herring	4.00
Wholemeal bread	4.10
Hovis	4.20
Wholemeal flour	5.70
Muesli	6.50
Topside of beef, cooked	6.50
Leg of lamb, cooked	6.60
Baked salmon	7.00
Roast chicken	8.20
Roast turkey	8.50
Boiled prawns	9.50
Peanuts	13.80
Cornflakes	16.00
Rice Krispies	16.00

Vitamin B6 – Pyridoxine
Milligrams per 100 g (3.5 oz)

Carrots	0.05
Full-fat milk	0.06
Skimmed milk	0.06
Semi-skimmed milk	0.06
Satsuma	0.07
White bread	0.07
White rice	0.07
Cabbage, boiled	0.08
Cottage cheese	0.08
Cox's apple	0.08
Wholemeal pasta	0.08
Frozen peas	0.09
Spinach, boiled	0.09
Cheddar cheese	0.10
Orange	0.10
Broccoli	0.11
Hovis	0.11
Baked beans	0.12
Boiled egg	0.12
Red kidney beans, cooked	0.12
Wholemeal bread	0.12
Tomatoes	0.14
Almonds	0.15
Cauliflower	0.15
Brussels sprouts	0.19
Sweetcorn, boiled	0.21
Leg of lamb, cooked	0.22
Grapefruit juice	0.23
Roast chicken	0.26
Lentils, boiled	0.28
Banana	0.29
Brazil nuts	0.31
Potatoes, boiled	0.32

Roast turkey	0.33	Eggs, whole, free-range	2.70
Grilled herring	0.33	Kambu seaweed	2.80
Topside of beef, cooked	0.33	Squid, frozen	2.90
Avocado	0.36	Taramasalata	2.90
Grilled cod	0.38	Duck, cooked	3.00
Baked salmon	0.57	Turkey, dark meat	3.00
Soya flour	0.57	Grapenuts	5.00
Hazelnuts	0.59	Tuna in oil	5.00
Peanuts	0.59	Herring, cooked	6.00
Walnuts	0.67	Herring roe, fried	6.00
Muesli	1.60	Steamed salmon	6.00
Cornflakes	1.80	Bovril	8.30
Rice Crispies	1.80	Mackerel, fried	10.00
Special K	2.20	Rabbit, stewed	10.00

Vitamin B12 – Cyanocobalamine

Micrograms per 100 g (3.5 oz)

Tempeh	0.10	Cod's roe, fried	11.00
Miso	0.20	Pilchards canned in tomato juice	12.00
Quorn	0.30	Oysters, raw	15.00
Full-fat mik	0.40	Nori seaweed	27.50
Skimmed milk	0.40	Sardines in oil	28.00
Semi-skimmed milk	0.40	Lamb's kidney, fried	79.00
Marmite	0.50		
Cottage cheese	0.70		
Choux buns	1.00		

Folate/Folic Acid

Micrograms per 100 g (3.5 oz)

Eggs, boiled	1.00	Cox's apple	4.00
Eggs, poached	1.00	Leg of lamb, cooked	4.00
Halibut, steamed	1.00	Full-fat milk	6.00
Lobster, boiled	1.00	Skimmed milk	6.00
Sponge cake	1.00	Semi-skimmed milk	6.00
Turkey, white meat	1.00	Porridge with semi-skimmed milk	7.00
Waffles	1.00	Turnip, baked	8.00
Cheddar cheese	1.20	Sweet potato, boiled	8.00
Eggs, scrambled	1.20	Cucumber	9.00
Squid	1.30	Grilled herring	10.00
Eggs, fried	1.60	Roast chicken	10.00
Shrimps, boiled	1.80	Avocado	11.00
Parmesan cheese	1.90	Grilled cod	12.00
Beef, lean	2.00	Banana	14.00
Cod, baked	2.00	Roast turkey	15.00
Cornflakes	2.00	Carrots	17.00
Pork, cooked	2.00	Sweet potato	17.00
Raw beef mince	2.00	Tomatoes	17.00
Rice Krispies	2.00	Topside of beef, cooked	17.00
Steak, lean, grilled	2.00	Swede, boiled	18.00
Edam cheese	2.10	Strawberries	20.00
Eggs, whole, battery	2.40	Brazil nuts	21.00
Milk, dried, whole	2.40	Red peppers, raw	21.00
Milk, dried, skimmed	2.60	Green peppers, raw	23.00
		Rye bread	24.00

Dates, fresh	25.00	Red kidney beans	1.00
New potatoes, boiled	25.00	Carrots	2.00
Grapefruit	26.00	Cucumber	2.00
Oatcakes	26.00	Muesli with dried fruit	2.00
Cottage cheese	27.00	Apricots, raw	6.00
Baked salmon	29.00	Avocado	6.00
Cabbage, boiled	29.00	Pear	6.00
Onions, boiled	29.00	Potato, boiled	6.00
White bread	29.00	Spinach, boiled	8.00
Orange	31.00	Cox's apple	9.00
Baked beans	33.00	Turnip	10.00
Cheddar cheese	33.00	Banana	11.00
Clementines	33.00	Frozen peas	12.00
Raspberries	33.00	Lamb's liver, fried	12.00
Satsuma	33.00	Pineapple	12.00
Blackberries	34.00	Dried skimmed milk	13.00
Rye crispbread	35.00	Gooseberries	14.00
Potato, baked in skin	36.00	Raw dates	14.00
Radish	38.00	Melon	17.00
Boiled egg	39.00	Tomatoes	17.00
Hovis	39.00	Cabbage, boiled	20.00
Wholemeal bread	39.00	Canteloupe melon	26.00
Red kidney beans, boiled	42.00	Cauliflower	27.00
Potato, baked	44.00	Satsuma	27.00
Frozen peas	47.00	Peach	31.00
Almonds	48.00	Raspberries	32.00
Parsnips, boiled	48.00	Bran flakes	35.00
Cauliflower	51.00	Grapefruit	36.00
Green beans, boiled	57.00	Mangoes	37.00
Broccoli	64.00	Nectarine	37.00
Walnuts	66.00	Kumquats	39.00
Artichoke	68.00	Broccoli	44.00
Hazelnuts	72.00	Lychees	45.00
Spinach, boiled	90.00	Unsweetened apple juice	49.00
Brussels sprouts	110.00	Orange	54.00
Peanuts	110.00	Kiwi fruit	59.00
Muesli	140.00	Brussels sprouts	60.00
Sweetcorn, boiled	150.00	Strawberries	77.00
Asparagus	155.00	Blackcurrants	115.00
Chickpeas	180.00		
Lamb's liver, fried	240.00		
Cornflakes	250.00		
Rice Krispies	250.00		
Calf's liver, fried	320.00		

Vitamin C
Milligrams per 100 g (3.5 oz)

Full-fat milk	1.00
Skimmed milk	1.00
Semi-skimmed milk	1.00

Vitamin D
Micrograms per 100 g (3.5 oz)

Skimmed milk	0.01
Whole milk	0.03
Fromage frais	0.05
Cheddar cheese	0.26
Cornflakes	2.80
Rice Krispies	2.80
Kellogg's Start	4.20
Margarine	8.00

Vitamin E
Milligrams per 100 g (3.5 oz)

Semi-skimmed milk	0.03
Boiled potatoes	0.06
Cucumber	0.07
Cottage cheese	0.08
Full-fat milk	0.09
Cabbage, boiled	0.10
Leg of lamb, cooked	0.10
Cauliflower	0.11
Roast chicken	0.11
Frozen peas	0.18
Red kidney beans, cooked	0.20
Wholemeal bread	0.20
Orange	0.24
Topside of beef, cooked	0.26
Banana	0.27
Brown rice, boiled	0.30
Grilled herring	0.30
Lamb's liver, fried	0.32
Baked beans	0.36
Cornflakes	0.40
Pear	0.50
Cheddar cheese	0.53
Carrots	0.56
Lettuce	0.57
Cox's apple	0.59
Grilled cod	0.59
Rice Krispies	0.60
Plums	0.61
Unsweetened orange juice	0.68
Leeks	0.78
Sweetcorn, boiled	0.88
Brussels sprouts	0.90
Broccoli	1.10
Boiled egg	1.11
Tomato	1.22
Watercress	1.46
Parsley	1.70
Spinach, boiled	1.71
Olives	1.99
Butter	2.00
Onions, dried raw	2.69
Mushrooms, fried in corn oil	2.84
Avocado	3.20
Muesli	3.20
Walnuts	3.85
Peanut butter	4.99
Olive oil	5.10
Sweet potato, baked	5.96
Brazil nuts	7.18
Peanuts	10.09
Pine nuts	13.65
Rapeseed oil	18.40
Almonds	23.96
Hazelnuts	24.98
Sunflower oil	48.70

Calcium
Milligrams per 100 g (3.5 oz)

Cox's apple	4.00
Brown rice, boiled	4.00
Potatoes, boiled	5.00
Banana	6.00
Topside of beef, cooked	6.00
White pasta, boiled	7.00
Tomato	7.00
White spaghetti, boiled	7.00
Leg of lamb, cooked	8.00
Red peppers, raw	8.00
Roast chicken	9.00
Roast turkey	9.00
Avocado	11.00
Pear	11.00
Butter	15.00
Cornflakes	15.00
White rice, boiled	18.00
Grilled cod	22.00
Lentils, boiled	22.00
Baked salmon	29.00
Green peppers, raw	30.00
Young carrots	30.00
Grilled herring	33.00
Wholemeal flour	38.00
Turnips, baked	45.00
Orange	47.00
Baked beans	48.00
Wholemeal bread	54.00
Boiled egg	57.00
Peanuts	60.00
Cottage cheese	73.00
Soya beans, boiled	83.00
White bread	100.00
Full-fat milk	115.00
Hovis	120.00
Muesli	120.00
Skimmed milk	120.00
Semi-skimmed milk	120.00
Prawns, boiled	150.00
Spinach, boiled	150.00
Brazil nuts	170.00
Yoghurt, low-fat, plain	190.00
Soya flour	210.00
Almonds	240.00

White self-raising flour	450.00
Sardines	550.00
Sprats, fried	710.00
Cheddar cheese	720.00
Whitebait, fried	860.00

Chromium

Micrograms per 100 g (3.5 oz)

Egg yolk	183.00
Molasses	121.00
Brewer's yeast	117.00
Beef	57.00
Hard cheese	56.00
Liver	55.00
Fruit juices	47.00
Wholemeal bread	42.00

Iron

Milligrams per 100 g (3.5 oz)

Semi-skimmed milk	0.05
Skimmed milk	0.06
Full-fat milk	0.06
Cottage cheese	0.10
Orange	0.10
Cox's apple	0.20
Pear	0.20
White rice	0.20
Banana	0.30
Cabbage, boiled	0.30
Cheddar cheese	0.30
Avocado	0.40
Grilled cod	0.40
Potatoes, boiled	0.40
Young carrots, boiled	0.40
Brown rice, boiled	0.50
Tomato	0.50
White pasta, boiled	0.50
Baked salmon	0.80
Roast chicken	0.80
Roast turkey	0.90
Grilled herring	1.00
Red peppers, raw	1.00
Boiled prawns	1.10
Green peppers, raw	1.20
Baked beans	1.40
Wholemeal spaghetti, boiled	1.40
White bread	1.60
Spinach, boiled	1.70
Boiled egg	1.90
White self-raising four	2.00
Brazil nuts	2.50
Peanuts	2.50

Leg of lamb, cooked	2.70
Wholemeal bread	2.70
Topside of beef, cooked	2.80
Almonds	3.00
Soya beans, boiled	3.00
Lentils, boiled	3.50
Hovis	3.70
Wholemeal flour	3.90
Muesli	5.60
Cornflakes	6.70
Rice Krispies	6.70
Soya flour	6.90

Magnesium

Milligrams per 100 g (3.5 oz)

Butter	2.00
Cox's apple	6.00
Turnip, baked	6.00
Young carrots	6.00
Tomato	7.00
Cottage cheese	9.00
Orange	10.00
Full-fat milk	11.00
White rice, boiled	11.00
Semi-skimmed milk	11.00
Skimmed milk	12.00
Boiled egg	12.00
Cornflakes	14.00
Potatoes, boiled	14.00
Red peppers, raw	14.00
White pasta, boiled	15.00
Wholemeal spaghetti, boiled	15.00
White self-raising flour	20.00
Green peppers, raw	24.00
Roast chicken	24.00
Topside of beef, cooked	24.00
White bread	24.00
Avocado	25.00
Cheddar cheese	25.00
Grilled cod	26.00
Roast turkey	27.00
Leg of lamb, cooked	28.00
Baked salmon	29.00
Baked beans	31.00
Spinach, boiled	31.00
Grilled herring	32.00
Banana	34.00
Lentils, boiled	34.00
Boiled prawns	42.00
Wholemeal spaghetti, boiled	42.00
Brown rice, boiled	43.00
Hovis	56.00

Soya beans, boiled	63.00
Wholemeal bread	76.00
Muesli	85.00
Wholemeal flour	120.00
Peanuts	210.00
Soya flour	240.00
Almonds	270.00
Brazil nuts	410.00

Selenium

Micrograms per 100 g (3.5 oz)

Full-fat milk	1.00
Semi-skimmed milk	1.00
Skimmed milk	1.00
Baked beans	2.00
Cornflakes	2.00
Orange	2.00
Peanuts	3.00
Almonds	4.00
Cottage cheese	4.00
White rice	4.00
White self-raising flour	4.00
Soya beans, boiled	5.00
Boiled egg	11.00
Cheddar cheese	12.00
White bread	28.00
Wholemeal bread	35.00
Lentils, boiled	40.00
Wholemeal flour	53.00

Zinc

Milligrams per 100 g (3.5 oz)

Butter	0.10
Pear	0.10
Orange	0.10
Red peppers, raw	0.10
Banana	0.20
Young carrots	0.20
Cornflakes	0.30
Potatoes, boiled	0.30
Avocado	0.40
Full-fat milk	0.40
Skimmed milk	0.40
Green peppers, raw	0.40
Semi-skimmed milk	0.40
Baked beans	0.50
Grilled cod	0.50
Grilled herring	0.50
White pasta	0.50
Tomatoes	0.50

Cottage cheese	0.60
Spinach, boiled	0.60
White bread	0.60
White self-raising flour	0.60
Brown rice	0.70
White rice	0.70
Soya beans, boiled	0.90
Wholemeal spaghetti, boiled	1.10
Boiled egg	1.30
Lentils, boiled	1.40
Roast chicken	1.50
Boiled prawns	1.60
Wholemeal bread	1.80
Hovis	2.10
Cheddar cheese	2.30
Roast turkey	2.40
Muesli	2.50
Wholemeal flour	2.90
Almonds	3.20
Peanuts	3.50
Brazil nuts	4.20
Leg of lamb, cooked	5.30
Topside of beef, cooked	5.50

Essential Fatty Acids

Exact amounts of these fats are hard to quantify. Good sources for the two families of essential fatty acids are given.

Omega-6 Series Essential Fatty Acids

Sunflower oil
Rapeseed oil
Corn oil
Almonds
Walnuts
Brazil nuts
Sunflower seeds
Soya products including tofu

Omega-3 Series Essential Fatty Acids

Mackerel ⎫
Herring ⎬ fresh cooked or
Salmon ⎭ smoked/pickled
Walnuts and walnut oil
Rapeseed oil
Soya products and soy bean oil

UK Directory of Soya Rich Foods

Soya Milks

So Good - Chilled
Alpro – Chilled
Plamil
Granose
Bonsoi
Sojasun
Ecomil

Smoothies & Shakes

Granose fruit shakes
Mangajo
Yofu Smoothies

Tofu

Dragonfly
Clearspot
Cauldron Foods
Full of Beans
Viana
Biona
Taifun

Tempeh

Full of Beans
Impulse Foods

Soya Bars

Wallaby bars

Soya Nuts

Clearspring Organic Roasted Snack Mix
Hearties (roasted nuts)

Ice Cream

Toffuti
Swedish Glace
Choices choc ices (Soya Health Foods)

Sunrise

Cream And Desserts

Soya Dream – Alpro
So Good Fruit Desserts
Alpro desserts - Vanilla and Chocolate
Granose Soya Cream

Flour

Planet Organic (own brand)
Goodness Foods
Doves Farm

Pastas

Orgran (rice and soya mix)

Yogurt

Alpro
Sojsdun

Soya And Linseed Loaf

Burgen Bread
Vogel's Soya & Linseed Loaf
Paul's Bakery - soya and brown rice

Cookies

Granny Ann Biscuits & Biscuit Cakes
Premier Harvest Chocolate Chip
Cookie Mix

Other Interesting Products

Tinned braised tofu (Marigold)
Realeat Vege Roast
Realeat Vege Mince
Realeat Vege Bacon
Marks & Spencer's range of foods containing soya
Safeway Vegetarian Lamb & Mint Style Steaks
Safeway Gammon Style Steaks

Australian Directory of Soya Rich Foods

Milks

So Natural
Vita Soya
Soya Life
Vita Life
Sanitarium
Sungold
Pure Harvest
Organic
Aussie Soya

Yoghurts & Smoothies

Sanitarium	**So Good Smoothie**
Soya Life	Yoghurt
So Natural	Yoghurt
King Land	Yoghurt
Soygurt	Yoghurt (organic)

Mayonnaises, Cheeses & Butters

King Land	**Mayo**
King Land	"Butter"
King Land	Soya Cheese
"Cheddar"	Simply Better
Foods	Soya Cheese
Organic	
Fine Quality Foods	Mayo
Norganic	Golden Soya Mayo

Ice Creams & Chocolates

Sweet William	**Soya Chocolate**
	Original
	Roasted Almond
	Rice Crackle

Sanitarium
Fruccio

So Good Ice Cream
Dairy Free Ice Cream

Tofu & Tempeh

TLY Joyce	**Tofu (Silken & Firm)**
Soyco	Tofu
Pureland	Tofu Organic
	Soya Star
Herb Tofu	
Nutri Soya	Tofu
King Land	Tofu Organic
Tally Ho Farm	Tempeh
	Tally Ho Farm
Seasoned Tofu	Beijing Soybean
Product	Tofu

Breads & Bread Mixes

Defiance	**Soya & Linseed Breadmix**
Clarona PTY "The Gluten Free Baker"	Maize & Soya Bread
Life's Harvest	Rye with Soya & Linseed Bread
Tip Top Burgen	Soya-Lin Bread
Helgas	Soya/Linseed Bread
Kitchen Collections	Soya & Linseed Breadmix

Cereals

Sanitarium	**Soya Tasty**
Lowan	Multiflakes with S & L
Uncle Tobys	Healthwise for Women 40+
Sun Sol	Soya Protein Muesli
Norganic	Soya Crunch
Vogels	Soya & Linseed Ultra Bran

Vogels	Soytana

Other Interesting Soya Products

Tally Ho Farm	**Soya Wedges**
Bon Vit	Powdered Soya Drink (Choc. Flavour)
Loose Chips	Soya Crisps and Various Flavours
Sun Sol	Linseed Meal
Sanitarium	Garlic & Herb Slices
Soya Healthy	Soya Sausages

Medical References:

1. Cruising Through The Menopause, Stewart, M. Vermilion, 2000

2. Rodriguez C et al. Oestrogen Replacement Therapy and Ovarian Cancer Mortality in a Large Prospective Study of U.S. Women. JAMA 2001; 285:1460-1465. Weiss NS, Rossing MA. Oestrogen-Replacement Therapy and Risk of Ovarian Cancer. The Lancet, 2001, vol. 358:438.

3. CSM/MCA Current Problems in Pharmacovigilance, October 2000: Vol. 28.

Schmidt PJ et al. Oestrogen replacement in perimenopause; related depression: A preliminary report. Am J Obstet. Gynecol.2000; 183:414-20.

5. Paola Albertazzi, et al, The Effect of Dietary Soya Supplementation on Hot Flushes. Obstetrics and Gynaecology, Vol. 91, No.1 January 1998 pp 6-11

6. The Role of Isoflavones in Menopausal Health: Consensus Opinion of the North American Menopause Society, Menopause: The Journal of the North American Menopause Society, Vol.7, No.4, pp 215-229

7. Nachtigall L, Journal of the British Menopause Society, Supplement S1 2001 pp 8-11

8. File, Sandra E et al. Eating soya improves human memory. Psychopharmacology (2001) 157:430-436

9. Nachtigall, LB, Nachtigall, MJ, Nachtigall, LE; Nonprescription Alternatives to Hormone Replacement Therapy; The Female Patient; June 1999; Vol 24: 45-50.

10. St Clair, R.W.; Oestrogens and atherosclerosis: phytoestrogens and selective oestrogen receptor modulators; Curr Opin Lipidol., 1998; 9(5):457-63.

11. Eden, J.; Phytoestrogens and the menopause; Baillière's Clinical Endocrinology and Metabolism, 1998; 12 (4): 581-87.

12. Adlercreutz, H & Mazur, W. (1997) Phyto-oestrogens and Western Diseases. The Finnish Medical Society DUODECIM, Annals of Medicine 29:95-120.

13. Mazur, W. Phytoestrogen content in foods. Baillière's Clinical Endocrinology & Metabolism 1998 Dec; 12(4): 729-42.

14. Tham, D et al. (1998) Potential Health Benefits of Dietary Phytoestrogens: A Review of the Clinical, Epidemiological, and Mechanistic Evidence. Journal of Clinical Endocrinology and Metabolism 83(7): 2223-2235.

15. Messina, M. Soyfoods and soybean phyto-oestrogens (isoflavones as possible alternatives to hormone replacement therapy (HRT). European Journal of Cancer 36 (2000) (S71-S72)

16. Messina, M. Messina V. Soyfoods, Soybean Isoflavones, and Bone Healthy: A Brief Overview. Journal of Renal Nutrition,

Vol 10, No 2 (April), 2000: pp 63, 68.

Le Blanc ES et al. Hormone Replacement Therapy and Cognition. JAMA 2001; 285: 1489-1499

Somekawa Y, et al, 'Soya intake related to Menopausal symptoms, serum lipids, and bone mineral density in postmenopausal Japanese Women', Obstetrics and Gynaecology, Vol.97, No.1, Jan 2001, pp 109-115

Alan Husband, Red Clover isoflavone supplements: safety and pharmacokinetics, Journal of the British Menopause Society, September S1, 2001, pp 4-7

The Role of Isoflavones in Menopausal Health: Consensus Opinion of the North American Menopause Society, Menopause: The Journal of the North American Menopause Society, Vol.7, No.4, pp 215-229

Nachtigall L, Journal of the British Menopause Society, Supplement S1 2001 pp 8-11.

Nagata C et al. Soya Product intake & hot flushes in Japanese women: Results from a community-based prospective study. Am J Eppidemiol 2001;153:790-3

Rice MM, et al. Tofu consumption and cognition in older Japanese American men and women. J. Nutr 2000' 130-676S.

Isoflavones from red clover (Promensil significantly reduce hot flushes compared with placebo. Van de Weijer PHM, Barensten R. Maturitas 2002; 187-193

The Use of an Isoflavone Supplement to Relive Hot Flushes in Postmenopausal Peruvian Women. Jeri AR. The Female Patient 2002; 27: 35-37

Phytoestrogens and Menopause AJ Husband. Br Med. J. 2002; 324:52

RECOMMENDED READING

Cruising Through the Menopause, Maryon Stewart, Vermilion

The Phyto Factor, Maryon Stewart, Vermilion

The Natural Health Bible, Maryon Stewart and Dr Alan Stewart, Vermilion

---

Address of the The Natural Health Advisory Service which incorporates the WNAS is:

PO Box 268, Lewes, East Sussex BN7 1YJ
Telephone: 01273 487366
Email: enquiries@naturalmenopause.com

Links to useful websites
www.beatmenopausenaturally.com
www.naturalhealthas.com

Mail Order Service for Books & Recommended Supplements
Recommended books and supplements can be obtained from the shop
at **www.beatmenopausenaturally.com** or by calling **0845 11 300 31**

Natural Health Advisory Service

MENOPAUSE SYMPTOMATOLOGY DIARY

Name: ....

GRADING OF **O** - None **1** - Mild-present but does not interfere with activities
SYMPTOMS **2** - Moderate - present and interferes with activities but not disabling
3 - Severe - disabling. Unable to function

DATE																									
MENSES																									
Hot/cold flushes																									
Facial/body flushing																									
Night sweats																									
Palpitations																									
Panic attacks																									
Generalised aches & pains																									
Depression																									
Perspiration																									
Numbness/skin tingling in arms/legs																									
Headaches																									
Backache																									
Fatigue																									
Irritability																									
Anxiety																									
Nervousness																									
Loss of confidence																									
Insomnia																									
Giddiness/dizziness																									
Difficulty/frequency in passing water																									
Constipation																									
Itchy vagina																									
Dry vagina																									
Painful intercourse																									
Decreased sex drive																									
Loss of concentration																									
Confusion/Loss of vitality																									
Water Retention																									
Bloated Abdomen																									
Weight in stones & pounds																									
Frequency of sexual intercourse (tick appropriate day)																									
Enjoyment of sexual intercourse (score between 0-10)																									

Additional Notes:

Natural Health Advisory Service

DIET DIARY

Name _____ Date _____

Address _____

Please complete on a daily basis for all food and drink consumed

	Breakfast	**Lunch**	**Dinner**	**Snacks**	**Excercise/ Supplements/ Symptoms**
Day 1					
Day 2					
Day 3					
Day 4					
Day 5					
Day 6					
Day 7					